MW01135694

RESCUED
BY THE U.S. COAST GUARD

RESCUED
BY THE U.S. COAST GUARD

GREAT ACTS
OF HEROISM
SINCE 1878

DENNIS L. NOBLE

NAVAL INSTITUTE PRESS
Annapolis, Maryland

Naval Institute Press
291 Wood Road
Annapolis, MD 21402

Library of Congress Cataloging-in-Publication Data
Noble, Dennis L.
Rescued by the U.S. Coast Guard : great acts of heroism since 1878 /
Dennis L. Noble.
    p. cm.
    Includes bibliographical references and index.
    ISBN 1-59114-625-9 (alk. paper)
    1. Lifesaving—United States—History. 2. United States. Coast
Guard—History. 3. Lifesaving stations—United States. I. Title.
VK1323.N6299 2004
363.28'6'0973—dc22

                                             2004019829

Printed in the United States of America on acid-free paper ∞
12 11 10 09 08 07 06 05   9 8 7 6 5 4 3 2
First printing

For Mark Ritten, A. J. Rose, Kevin Schutte, Lee Seckinger,
and all those who try to save others at sea—
past, present, and future.

There were times that the only thing that kept us from turning back because we were so cold, sick, and miserable was that we were too damned scared to realize we were all of those other things.

———

Cdr. Michael C. Monteith, former commanding officer,
U.S. Coast Guard Station Cape Disappointment, Washington

Contents

Preface

This book is about people who put themselves into harm's way for others. I decided to undertake it after writing two previous books dealing with the U.S. Coast Guard's maritime search and rescue (SAR). Research reveals that most Americans know very little about the U.S. Coast Guard—except for SAR. Sebastian Junger, in his best-selling book *The Perfect Storm,* said it best: "Any weekend boater knows the Coast Guard will pluck him out of whatever idiocy he gets himself into."

The public affairs office of the service constantly hammers this point. In April 2003, for example, U.S. Coast Guard headquarters said that on an average day the service conducts 109 SAR cases, saves 10 lives, and helps 192 people in distress. A closer look at some statistics indicates that public affairs is not dealing in the normal government hyperbole. The Thirteenth Coast Guard District's public affairs office, for example, said that for one year in the coastal Washington-Oregon area, U.S. Coast Guard crews saved three hundred people and conducted 2,795 SAR cases. Other districts make similar claims. Truly an impressive record.

The record of rescues by the U.S. Coast Guard and its predecessor agency, the U.S. Life-Saving Service, appears a treasure trove for anyone wishing to write on maritime SAR. Amazingly, one of the most difficult subjects for a writer to explore concerning the U.S. Coast Guard is rescue after 1915. For some inexplicable reason, the leadership of the service since that time has failed to see any reason to publicize the work of their crews. Just as bad, the leadership since the end of World War II has failed to preserve the records of rescues for others to use. Researchers constantly hear the "We are unable to locate any records" refrain from district public affairs offices. Many districts do not even reply to requests for information on rescues. Little wonder that few books are written on the history of SAR in the service. Although the service has a history office, the leadership has seldom seen the value of passing on to that office the paperwork concerning rescues for which crews received high awards. Very few public affairs offices have seen the value of interviewing the people who received high medals for bravery and passing these interviews on to the service's history office.

The leadership's seeming indifference to rescues is even more glaring when it comes to the lack of information on the people who perform rescues. Since 1915, there have been only two books, one published by a commercial publisher and one by an academic press, that examined the people who serve at the service's small boat stations. Nor has the aviation branch of the service received much credit. Only one book by a New York publisher has examined rescue-by-helicopter crews in depth. To date, there has been no book-length biography by a commercial publisher of any person whose career focused on SAR. There has been one self-published autobiography. This despite the fact that since 1918 there were seventy-nine incidents for which rescuers received the Gold Life Saving Medal.

In 2000, I made a request to U.S. Coast Guard Headquarters for a listing of those awarded the Coast Guard Medal, the highest medal awarded personnel at the service's small boat rescue stations for valor in peacetime. Headquarters provided a listing of the people, but not their citations or any photographs of them or, often, the stations from which the rescue occurred. Headquarters discarded the citations. In other words, the U.S. Coast Guard knew it had heroes but did not know what they had accomplished. It was a civilian interested in the history of the Coast Guard Medal who made research into the medal and those who received it possible. He graciously turned over the information on citations he had amassed to the historian's office. It is hoped that the rescue cases in this book will give a glimpse of some of the people who work in SAR and help erase the anonymity.

This book has two purposes. One is to gather what material is available and present a nationwide look at the U.S. Coast Guard's rescues from shore-based stations from 1878 to 2003. The second is to give readers a look at the men and women who are at the leading edge of the service's SAR program. To understand both rescues and the people who perform them, it is necessary to give an overview of how rescue equipment has evolved over the years, but discussions on equipment are only overviews.

While most of the rescues selected for this book are those for which men and women received high awards, a majority of those serving in the U.S. Coast Guard will never be involved in a high-profile case. They do their everyday work and respond to calls for towing or medical assistance. Because there is such a paucity of material on the people and routines at the various units, it is difficult to convey to those who have no notion of maritime SAR that not everyone wins medals. If most Americans could read all the cases performed by those in SAR, they quickly would grasp that even "routine" cases are often not routine. Again, the lack of records, newspaper accounts, and so forth greatly narrowed the selection process. Despite tales from old salts, or the finding of citations, some exciting stories are not in this book because of a lack of supporting material.

Whenever possible, especially for more recent rescues, I have let the people involved in a rescue describe the event. In those accounts based on interviews, very little has been edited from the transcripts, only the false starts and repetitions found in normal speech patterns. Although some accounts may not be grammatically correct, it is how the people involved remembered their experiences and it is important for readers to see the scene as the lifesavers viewed it.

I divided the book into four parts roughly corresponding to the development of the lifeboat and the motor lifeboat, the heavy weather boat of the service. As rescue by small boat is the service's most historic method, this seemed the best way to measure the changing face of SAR within the U.S. Coast Guard.

I admit to a bias toward the small boat stations. Statistics prove that they conduct the majority of SAR in the service. Concentrating solely on the stations, however, does not give a true picture of maritime SAR. To give a broader view, I also describe rescues undertaken by air stations and a patrol boat.

If this book helps Americans better understand the people who have served so faithfully for so many years, and if it helps people understand some of the amazing rescues the lifesavers have accomplished over the years, then it will have accomplished its purpose.

My first published account of SAR in the U.S. Coast Guard appeared more than thirty years ago. During the last seven years, I have visited many stations throughout the United States to gain firsthand insight into the work of the people who conduct SAR. Over these years, crews have never failed to readily provide me with information and insights into their world. Most have made me, an outsider, feel I was a member of a crew—a high honor, indeed. I finished this book in stages at the following stations located near my home: Neah Bay, Washington; Quillayute River, Washington; Gray's Harbor, Washington; Cape Disappointment, Washington; Tillamook Bay, Oregon; Yaquina Bay, Oregon; Umpqua River, Oregon; and Coos Bay, Oregon.

Acknowledgments

oet John Donne wrote, "No man is an island, entire of itself." I could not tell the story of the U.S. Coast Guard's rescues without the help of many people. Some are not mentioned in the acknowledgments but appear in the notes.

I am most indebted to Dr. Robert M. Browning Jr., Historian of the U.S. Coast Guard, and his staff, Scott Price and Christopher Havern, at U.S. Coast Guard Headquarters. They quickly responded to my many requests and made research much easier. All researchers should have such professional help.

The following U.S. Coast Guard personnel provided me with a great deal of information and other assistance: BMCM Stephen Bielman, Lt. Richard J. Burke Jr., ASM 1st Class Charles Carter, BMC Jerry Farmer, BMC Aaron Ferguson, Lt. C.A. Ferguson, BMC Jon Gagnon, Lt. William Gibbons, CWO4 Richard W. Glasgow, Capt. Dana Goward, CWO2 Michael Hoig, BMCM Lars Kent, CWO3 Richard Loser, Lt. Cdr. Daniel Johnson, Cdr. Paul A. Langlois, BMC Michael Mahoney, Cdr. Raymond J. Miller, BMC Wes Parker, Capt. William W. Peterson, Lt. Daniel Pickles, BMC Michael Saindon, Lt. Craig Sanders, BMCM William Sheretz, Lt.

Antonio Soltz; CWO3 James Stoffer, CWO4 Kenneth D. Stuber, BMC Shawn Vandrenburg, CWO2 Darrin Wallace, Capt. W. Russell Webster, and Lt. Michael F. White. I especially wish to thank all the crews who made me feel welcome and provided so much information on their lives.

Truman R. Strobridge, former Historian of the U.S. Coast Guard, read portions of the manuscript and checked to see whether I continued to use the past tense. Again, William "Bill" Wilkinson, Director Emeritus of the Mariner's Museum, willingly shared his vast amount of knowledge about the rescue craft of the U.S. Coast Guard. John Galluzzo, editor of *Wreck & Rescue,* helped locate material and shared his knowledge of the Cape Cod region. David Pearson of the Columbia River Maritime Museum was very helpful. Maritime Historian Frederick Stonehouse graciously supplied me with information and shared his expertise on shipwrecks on Lake Superior; Mary Sicchio, of the Cape Cod Community College, provided me with the photograph that depicts Bernard Webber after the amazing *Pendelton* rescue. Anne Kifer, secretary for the Association for Rescue at Sea, even though recovering from a bout of the flu, quickly responded to my request for information. Richard Schaefer at U.S. Coast Guard Headquarters provided me with statistics.

Readers and editors should appreciate the efforts of people who volunteered to read the manuscript, thus greatly improving it. Loren A. Noble not only read and commented upon the whole manuscript but also had to put up with my constant harping and pouting when things went wrong. Peggy Norris, once again, did her normal outstanding job of spotting my inconsistencies and misspellings. Greg Shield went above and beyond the call of duty. Despite a bad back, he dived into the manuscript and rescued me from mistakes.

At the Naval Institute Press, I thank Eric Mills, acquisitions editor, for seeing value in the work. Karin Kaufman's copyediting made the book read much better. The production editors successfully guided the book to completion.

The writing of this book was an experience akin to being locked in the forward compartment of a motor lifeboat in twenty-foot seas. I could not have finished without the help of all those mentioned above, and of many who go unmentioned, who, I hope, will excuse the oversight. Where the book has merit, it is because I listened to all of the people who helped me. Where the book falters, it is because I ignored their advice.

RESCUED
BY THE U.S. COAST GUARD

PART I
1878–1914

1 | Brave and Persistent Efforts

Maritime rescue from the shore has been a tradition in this country since the first shouts of "Ship ashore!" echoed along the beach. The early economy of the United States depended heavily upon maritime trade. In the age of sail, once a ship came upon soundings, it entered the most hazardous period of its voyage. Take, for example, the approach to busy nineteenth-century New York City's harbor.

A captain of a nineteenth-century sailing ship faced a gauntlet-like approach to the port of New York. The coast of New Jersey loomed on one side and Long Island, New York, on the other. During a strong nor'easter, New Jersey's shoreline became a lee shore. Both coasts contain sandbars located some three hundred to eight hundred yards offshore. In a gale, many ships quickly went to pieces when they struck the sandbars and were then pounded relentlessly by the surf. Few of their crews and passengers could survive the long swim to shore in forty-degree Fahrenheit storm-tossed seas. The few sailors or passengers who managed to stagger ashore in winter stood a good chance of perishing due to exposure on the largely uninhabited beaches. On 1 January 1837, for example, the emigrant packet *Mexico,* with 112 passengers and crew, ran into a strong storm within sight of the New Jersey coast. Capt. Charles Winslow ordered distress signals fired.[1]

Would-be rescuers on shore spotted the distress signals, but the violent sea made most hesitate. Toward dawn the seas began building to ever greater heights. *Mexico* started to drift hopelessly toward shore. At 5:00 A.M. on 2 January 1837, it struck heavily at what is now Long Beach, New York. Only a few onlookers tried to fight the seas. All on board *Mexico* were lost.[2]

This portion of the country's coast was not the only dangerous spot. The coastline from Maine to North Carolina presented great danger to mariners. As trade increased, there arose a greater need to provide help for ships wrecked close to shore.

Organized assistance to shipwrecked mariners from shore stations in this country began with volunteer lifesaving services, such as the Massachusetts Humane Society, in the late eighteenth century. A sailing ship trying to help near the shore also stood a good chance of running aground, especially if there were heavy onshore winds. Technology from the eighteenth century until the second decade of the twentieth century decreed that only small boats could help those close to the beach and out of range of any line-throwing device. The Massachusetts Humane Society founded the first life boat station at Cohassett, Massachusetts, in 1807. The society's stations consisted of small shedlike structures that held the volunteers' rescue equipment. Many of the first stations stood near the entrance to busy ports, thus leaving most of the coastline unprotected.[3]

In 1848, the federal government entered the shore-based life-saving business. New Jersey congressman William A. Newell made a successful appeal to Congress for ten thousand dollars to provide "surfboats, rockets, carronades and other necessary apparatus for the better preservation of life and property from shipwrecks on the coasts of New Jersey." The Massachusetts Humane Society also requested, and received, funds for establishing additional stations. Within the federal government, stations fell under the control of the Treasury Department through the Revenue Marine Bureau (later called the U.S. Revenue Cutter Service). Once established, the stations operated like volunteer fire departments, but without any provisions for supervision or inspection.[4]

The system of volunteers continued to expand for six years. When a strong storm swept the East Coast in 1854, many ship-wrecked people lost their lives because of a lack of stations or because the equipment in the existing ones had not been kept in condition for immediate use. One town, for example, used its life boat alternatively as a trough for mixing mortar and a tub for scalding hogs.[5]

Again, goaded by public outcry, Congress appropriated more funds for the stations, earmarking some of the money to employ a full-time keeper at each station and hire superintendents to over-see the units along the coasts of New Jersey and Long Island. Yet the problems continued. As one old waterman recalled, the only person on duty at a station was a keeper, and if he discovered a vessel in distress, he then had to search for a volunteer crew. Along the "wilds" of New Jersey's coast, the keeper could tramp for miles before rounding up a crew, and by that time the sailors and passengers aboard a wreck might be beyond help.[6]

The Civil War spelled a period of complete neglect of the sta-tions, which continued even after the ending of the war. In 1870, another disastrous storm swept the eastern seaboard. Newspaper editors called for reform to "check the terrible fatalities off our dangerous coasts" and revamp the lifesaving system so that mariners could depend upon help in the future.[7]

The year 1871 is an important date in the history of shore-based maritime rescue in this country. That year, Sumner Increase Kimball, a lawyer from Maine and a longtime Treasury employee, took over the reins of the Revenue Marine Bureau within the Treasury Department. The system of lifesaving stations came under his control. Soon after taking over his new duties, Kimball ordered Capt. John Faunce of the U.S. Revenue Marine to investi-gate the stations. Faunce found that their equipment was "rusty for want of care and some of it ruined," that some keepers were too old and others lived too far from the stations, and that a few keep-ers were incompetent for their positions. "Politics had had more influence in their appointment than qualification" for handling boats, he noted.[8]

Armed with Faunce's report, Kimball, the ultimate bureaucrat, went before Congress and received, for the time, the huge sum of two hundred thousand dollars to revamp the stations. Using his administrative skills, he set about reorganizing the system of lifesaving stations. He made the entire crew of a station a paid team subject to discipline and appointed inspectors from the Revenue Marine to check the stations periodically for efficiency. Kimball weeded out political appointees and those too old to perform their jobs. The crews showed gradual improvement, although there were still serious losses, such as those caused by the wrecks of the *Huron* and *Metropolis* along the Outer Banks of North Carolina in 1877 and 1878 that killed at least 183 people.[9]

When Kimball set about improving the stations, he convinced Congress to establish two medals for those who exhibited extraordinary valor in rescuing people from drowning. He succeeded in having the Gold and Silver Life Saving Medals established, the Gold being the senior award. These two medals are the oldest and among the most prestigious awards of the U.S. Coast Guard.

Kimball's efforts paid off. Soon, accounts of daring rescues began to appear in newspapers and magazines. The number of stations increased. In 1874, the stations expanded to include the coast of Maine and ten locations south of Cape Henry, Virginia, including the Outer Banks of North Carolina. The following year, the network expanded to include the Delaware-Maryland-Virginia peninsula, the Great Lakes, and the coast of Florida. Eventually, stations appeared at locations along the Gulf of Mexico and the West Coast. Even far-off Alaska received a unit at Nome.[10]

In 1878, the growing network of lifesaving stations became a separate agency of the Treasury Department and was named the U.S. Life-Saving Service. Not surprisingly, Sumner I. Kimball was named general superintendent of the service. He held tight control over the organization and remained its only general superintendent. The law that created the U.S. Coast Guard in 1915, by amalgamating the U.S. Revenue Cutter Service with the U.S. Life-Saving

Service, also provided for Kimball's retirement. The service's reputation for honest, efficient, and nonpartisan administration, and performance of duty, is the result of the efforts of this one man.[11]

CANNONS THAT SAVED LIVES

Lifesavers had two methods of rescuing people in distress. The most complicated involved establishing a strong rope bridge from the beach to the shipwreck. This required a line-throwing device. The operational range of the cannon was approximately six hundred yards. Once those on board the ship received the messenger line, they began to pull over stronger lines, until the heavy hawser came on board.[12]

Once the lifesavers successfully rigged the hawser, they then had two devices to bring people ashore. The first, a breeches buoy, resembled a life ring with canvas trousers. It moved out to the wreck along the hawser. A survivor climbed into the device and the lifesavers pulled the shipwrecked person ashore. The second device was the lifecar, also known as the surfcar, which resembled a small enclosed boat. Shipwrecked people entered the lifecar through a hatch (door). Once inside, the hatch tightly secured, lifesavers pulled the device along the hawser to safety. Usually only one to three people went inside the lifecar at a time, although it supposedly could hold eleven people for three minutes. It is hard to imagine eleven people in such a small contraption, but as one old waterman correctly put it, "Men in that extremity are not apt to stand on the order of their going." By the 1880s, the lifecar had fallen into disuse. It required an extra cart to bring it to the site, which taxed the resources of the small crews.[13]

The lifesavers stowed the breeches buoy, Lyle gun, powder, lines, and other paraphernalia on a cart known as the "beach apparatus" or "beach cart." They either pulled the cart themselves or hitched a horse to it. The beach apparatus was the most complicated means of rescue for the lifesavers. One of the changes that Kimball implemented in his reorganization, which today seems elementary, was the notion that crews needed to practice continually with all the weapons in their arsenal. Crews drilled, or practiced, each day of the week, except Sunday. Mondays and Thursdays crews drilled with the beach apparatus. On those days, the life-savers had to haul out the beach cart, set up the equipment, fire the Lyle gun, rig the hawser, and send out the breeches buoy. Finally, with a crewman pulled "ashore," the drill ended. For drills, each station had a drill pole in the shape of a mast. When inspectors came to the stations to test the units, the entire drill had to be completed within five minutes. Failure to finish the drill in time meant dismissal for those slowing the practice.[14]

The seemingly endless drills paid dividends. Trained surfmen could set up the equipment quickly and with little confusion. Drills also built confidence, which was vital. In howling winds on a stormy night, with the surf pounding on the beach, the temperature hovering near the freezing point, and the shotline fouled, it took great self-discipline and confidence to retrieve the equipment calmly and start over. The nearly rote performance of duty could be crucial, especially if the men were tired, wet, and cold from earlier work. Self-discipline, confidence, and leadership all came together during the rescue of *George Taulane* in 1880.

HEROISM ON A COLD BEACH

The schooner *George Taulane,* bound for New York from Virginia on 3 February 1880 with a deck cargo of cordwood and a crew of seven men, ran into a snowstorm before reaching Sandy Hook, New Jersey. Before attempting the tricky passage into New York's harbor, the captain, a wise seaman, ordered the crew to keep *Taulane* offshore in fifteen fathoms of water until the storm passed. Gradually, the wind increased until it reached gale intensity. As the schooner labored heavily, the skipper ordered the mainsail double reefed. At two o'clock in the morning, the deck cargo shifted and broke free. The hapless crew, in trying to secure the cargo, fought a plunging, heaving ship and had to dodge the large billets of wood sliding threateningly across the deck. As serious as this was, the winter night was not yet finished with *Taulane.*[15]

The cry dreaded by all sailors at sea rang out from the fore-castle: "Fire!" Flames, fanned by the raging wind, swept quickly through the deck cargo. If the crew could not control the fire, they would have to abandon ship, which meant certain death in the frigid, tossing seas. Somehow the small crew managed to control the fire. But with all hands engaged in fighting the blaze, the schooner drifted, slowly and inexorably, toward the beach.

Six hours after the crew of *George Taulane* had begun their struggles with fire, wind, and water, they saw in the dim, sleet-filled dawn the beach no more than one mile away. The skipper, thinking he could save the ship, let go both anchors in an attempt to hold it. But the elements still were not yet done with the schooner. A combination of a strong south current and gale-force winds proved too much for *Taulane*'s anchors, and they began to drag. The ship, now in the trough of the sea, took powerful broadsides from the raging storm. *Taulane* was rolling heavily, the seas "making clean breaches over her, staving and rendering, and sweeping everything off her deck"; the sailors were unable to cut the anchor cables. Instead, they managed "to scramble aloft for their lives." Three of them sought safety in the fore rigging, while the remainder scrambled up the main rigging.

With decks completely awash, the ship gradually began to close the beach, and it appeared the sea was about to claim more lives. Then *Taulane*'s crew spotted the lifesaving crew of Station 11 (Swan Point) following the schooner along the beach. The captain afterward said that "seeing this determined squad gave new life to [my] . . . despairing men."

The crew of the station at Swan Point had earlier spied *Taulane* approaching the shore. When it dropped its anchors, Keeper James Numan thought the schooner would drag in such a storm and ground closer to Station 12 (Green Island). The keeper then took a gamble: rather than pull the heavy beach apparatus, he ordered his men to grab only heaving lines and start after the drifting ship. Numan counted on the crew of Green Island to turn out with their cart when they spied the ship. Thus two crews would be on the scene and Numan's surfmen would not be worn out from hauling the heavy beach apparatus. The strategy paid off. The beach patrol of Green Island sighted *Taulane* and ran back to report to Keeper William P. Chadwick, who immediately ordered out his crew with the beach cart.

That cold February night's weather brought many unusual hazards. The tide was four feet higher than normal and the pounding surf surged up to the dune line. Surges cut sluices into the beach, and the sea rushed with uncontrolled energy into these cuts. Seas in the sluices generated enough force to sweep a man off his feet. The beach itself was another hazard. High water caused the sand to turn to the consistency of quicksand. In addition, the deck cargo of lumber and pieces of *Taulane* itself became deadly missiles when hurled ashore by the sea.

Station 12's surfmen began moving the beach apparatus in the direction of *Taulane*. The soft condition of the beach made it necessary for the lifesavers to push and pull the cart by hand for about a quarter of a mile. While the surfmen struggled with the apparatus, Keeper Chadwick gathered a team of horses and met his crew where the beach sand would finally support horses. Quickly hitched to the apparatus, the horses pulled steadily for at least a mile, but when the lifesavers reached a deep sluiceway, the horses balked. The surfmen grabbed the hauling ropes and pulled the cart through waist-deep water while keeping a wary eye out for hurling debris and trying to keep their footing. The horses, without their load, allowed the lifesavers to lead them across the sluiceway. On the other side, with the horses again hitched to the apparatus, the trek continued until halted by yet another sluiceway. Again, the men went into the water. From this point on, because the water was "so deep and the sand cut away so fast under the wheels," the surfmen abandoned the horses and pulled the cart themselves until they came abreast of *Taulane*. The two lifesaving crews finally met. Chadwick had managed to find six civilian volunteers to help his crew; nineteen men would now attempt the rescue. The hardship the rescuers had endured in just reaching *Taulane* was merely a prelude to what was in store for them. In the words of the U.S. Life-Saving Service, the nineteen lifesavers now entered into "a singular and memorable struggle."

Four hundred yards off shore, *Taulane* wallowed heavily, its hull almost underwater. Seven crewmen could be seen still clinging to the ratlines; one of them was hanging by his arms over a ratline with one leg through below.

The rescuers placed the Lyle gun atop a small sand hill. It was readied, aimed, and fired. The projectile and shotline flew across the flying jib stay, but the sailors on board *Taulane* could not reach it, and the men on shore hauled the line and projectile back. In the grip of the surf, the schooner surged farther to the south.

The nineteen-man rescue party put everything back onto the beach apparatus cart and hurried after the drifting schooner. Again the rescuers set up the Lyle gun. This time the shot fell short. The additional weight of the wet line shortened the range of the projectile. Again, the cart was loaded and the rescuers splashed and staggered with their burden four hundred yards down the beach. Automatically, the lifesavers unloaded the gun from the cart, reloaded it with black powder, and fired. This time the shotline broke, and the men resumed their exhausting chase after the moving schooner.

By now the wheels of the cart had "sanded down," that is, the wheels sunk deep into the wet, soft sand. To prevent the cart from being completely mired, the rescuers had to keep the apparatus in constant motion. To make better progress, only part of the equipment came off the cart; the lifesavers themselves carried the remaining gear. Men "would . . . fling themselves upon the wheels and hold them with all their strength to prevent the cart from being capsized" in the raging surf. Missile-like debris from *Taulane* struck the lifesavers. A piece of debris struck Chadwick so hard that his right arm was still "lame four months later."

The rescuers chased *Taulane*, unloaded the cart for the third time, and set up the Lyle gun, only to have the ship drift out of range again. The crews unloaded and loaded the gun from the cart at "least a dozen times" without getting off a shot. The schooner drifted past Station 12; about a quarter of a mile beyond the station, the rescuers saw a chance to fire. Again, however, the wet shotline parted. By now, the lifesavers and volunteers had been at it for nearly four hours. As the frustrated rescuers retrieved the remnants of the shotline, they saw a sailor from *Taulane*'s forward rigging fall to his death in the churning seas. Half an hour later, another man dropped from the rigging.

Staggering and floundering onward, spurred by the knowledge that to stop meant certain death for the sailors on *Taulane*, the lifesavers received another setback. A surge upset the cart and the Lyle gun went into over four feet of frigid seawater. The men groped in the numbing water for Lyle gun, the only instrument that could save the men aboard *Taulane*. A lifesaver found the gun and wiped it dry. Amazingly, after hours of exertion, one of the keepers—it is not clear which one—hoisted the 165-pound gun onto his shoulder and continued down the beach.

One surfman received orders from his keeper to run back to Station 12 for dry shotline. As he hurried to carry out his assignment, he heard the fifth shot of the night, but again the line parted. Once again, the keeper heaved the gun onto his shoulder and continued down the beach. The surfman returned with the dry line just in time; *Taulane* suddenly struck a north-setting tide, which stopped it and swung its bow offshore. "The time had come at last."

The lifesavers by now were numb from exhaustion and exposure. But the long hours of monotonous drill paid off as they instinctively set up for another shot. Quickly bending the dry shotline to the projectile, the keeper aimed the Lyle gun and yanked the firing lanyard. This time the projectile and shotline reached *Taulane*. Surfmen and volunteers rapidly rigged the apparatus. The sailors aboard *Taulane* grabbed the shotline and pulled the hawser out to the ship. Quickly, the breeches buoy followed. After the first two rescued sailors came ashore, the schooner grounded, increasing its rolling. The ship rolled so wildly that once the breeches buoy, with a sailor in it, swung "fully fifty feet in the air." Even with this carnival-like ride, the last man off the schooner reached safety just thirty minutes after the sailors were able to grab the shotline.

The U.S. Life-Saving Service's official report on the wreck of *Taulane* notes that the rescuers pursued the ship at least three miles and the entire rescue took "not less than six hours." The nineteen rescuers deservedly received the Gold Life Saving Medal.

THREE RESCUES IN CLEVELAND'S HARBOR

Beginning on Halloween 1883, more than three years after the wreck of *Taulane,* a series of rescues played out in the harbor of Cleveland, Ohio. Fighting a severe northwest gale, the three-masted schooner *Sophia Minch* attempted to gain the shelter of the harbor. *Minch* began its run into the harbor about seven in the evening, but heavy pounding disabled its rudder, obliging the skipper of the schooner to drop anchor and signal for assistance. The keeper of the Cleveland U.S. Life-Saving Service Station convinced the master of the tug *Peter Smith* to take two of his crew aboard his vessel to assist *Minch*. When they came alongside, *Minch*'s captain refused to heave up the anchor until more tugs arrived. The tug's captain returned to the harbor to seek the help from the tug *Fanny Tuthill*. Keeper Goodwin gathered the remainder of his crew and boarded *Smith* as it again steamed out to assist *Sophia Minch*. After some dangerous maneuvering, the lifesaving crew managed to scramble on board *Minch*. Surfman Lawrence Distel remained with *Smith* to handle lines. As the two tugs started pulling the ship toward the breakwater, both towlines parted in the heavy seas and the tugs retreated to safety.[16]

By now the seas had built to great heights and mountainous waves were breaking over *Minch,* filling its hold and dragging it toward the rocky shore. *Minch*'s captain decided to scuttle his ship. All hands now tried to escape the breaching seas in the rigging. The crashing waves, however, cut off two sailors, who huddled nervously in the mizzen rigging.

Meanwhile, the tug *Peter Smith* landed Surfman Distel on shore. Seeing the plight of his shipmates, Distel immediately began to seek volunteers to aid in their rescue. Not surprisingly, at two o'clock in the morning few were willing to turn out in the face of such a storm. At last only five men—Custom Inspector Bates, three civilians (Pryor, Duffy, and Tovat), and George Tower, the lighthouse keeper—volunteered to help.[17] Tovat supplied a team of horses to draw the beach apparatus cart, and soon the Lyle gun roared.

In a short time the breeches buoy had safely landed all the sailors from *Minch* except for two stranded in the mizzen rigging. Surfman Frederick T. Hatch remained aboard to help in their rescue, and Distel rode back across the storm-tossed waters in the breeches buoy to meet with Hatch to lay out a plan of action. The surfmen agreed that if Hatch failed to return in a reasonable time, Distel should make for the shore. With the main boom and gaff sweeping back and forth across the main deck, Surfman Hatch set off, dodging both stormy seas and tackle, to reach the stranded sailors. Miraculously, he made it aft and found both men safe, but the surfman knew that a return trip would be impossible.

Surfman Distel, true to the plan, had given the signal to return to shore. Once there, the lifesavers hauled in the gear. Now Keeper Goodwin had to place another shot near the location of Hatch and the two shipwrecked sailors. Goodwin aimed and fired another successful shot to *Minch*. In short order the sailors were ashore, Hatch being the sixteenth and last man to reach safety.

Keeper Goodwin and his crew may have thought they had earned some well-deserved rest after this ordeal, but the next day *John B. Merrill*, of Milwaukee, Wisconsin, wrecked near the site of *Minch*. The lifesavers quickly set up their apparatus, and in the stormy night the projectile flew to the ship. Everything went smoothly, and after securing the hawser, Surfman Hatch volunteered to go out to *Merrill* and help the sailors ashore. Within forty-five minutes the crew of ten was safely ashore.

Ten days after the rescue of the crew of *Merrill*, another strong storm, this time from the northwest, swept Lake Erie. At 7:30 P.M. on 11 November, the wind shifted to the northwest and, in the words of the official report of the U.S. Life-Saving Service, began blowing "a perfect hurricane." Keeper Goodwin had a surfman keep an alert lookout as ships began to run for shelter in the harbor. At 9:10, the schooner rigged barge *John T. Johnson* hove into sight, running before the wind under its mainsail and fore staysail. The storm had carried away its foreboom and threatened to sink the barge. *Johnson*'s skipper tried to make the lee of the breakwater but failed and ordered the anchor dropped opposite the east pier, about two hundred yards off the pier.

Keeper Goodwin, seeing the plight of *Johnson,* ordered his crew into the surfboat. Towering seas, however, prevented the lifesavers from clearing the breakwater. The captain of the tug *Forest City* came alongside and promised that if the lifesavers could get aboard *Johnson* and ship its anchors, he would try to tow her inside.

With great effort, the lifesavers finally managed to get their boat outside the breakwater, and using superb seamanship, Goodwin put his boat alongside *Johnson*. Some lifesavers scrambled up the side and tied off the boat. The waves broke over Goodwin and those of his crew who had remained in the boat. Water drenched the lifesavers and froze to ice when it struck the crew. Goodwin then signaled to the Customs House officer and lighthouse keeper to send a tug out. The tugs by this time, including *Forrest City,* "were afraid to venture out." Keeper Goodwin, with the broken promise of the tug's captain, knew he had to climb back into the small boat and make the difficult and dangerous trip to shore. Because *Johnson* still was under way, Goodwin could only wait on shore to see where the barge would ground. Once it grounded, lifesavers and volunteers could try to help its crew when it came ashore. Goodwin ordered Surfman John Eveleigh to remain aboard the barge to handle the lines of the beach apparatus.

The remainder of the lifesaving crew scrambled over the side into their boat. Goodwin felt it too dangerous to have *Johnson*'s crew in the boat. Events would prove that Goodwin, again, knew his profession. The boat shoved off. Within one hundred feet of the barge, the lifesaver's boat was half-filled with the frigid lake water breaking over the small craft. The boat's headway was checked. Goodwin knew the only chance they had was to quickly beach the boat, but the nearest beach for three miles was only 150 feet wide and too close to the Lake Shore Freight Piers. If the boat went under them, it meant "certain death."

Keeper Goodwin, using his steering sweep oar, and with his exhausted lifesavers at their oars, maneuvered the surfboat for an open beach landing in heavy weather, one of the most difficult and dangerous tasks in handling a small craft. At a distance of 150 yards of the beach, the boat turned sideways to the waves, broached, and capsized, flinging the crew into the icy waters. It was impossible to right the boat. The lifesavers were washed away from their craft. As the men struggled back to the boat, they were again flung away. Even with adrenaline now at full flow, the lifesaver's strength quickly ebbed. Wave after wave washed over the struggling men.

Meanwhile, a large, excited crowd had gathered on the pier. Many were sure they were witnessing the beginnings of a tragedy. Without thinking, onlookers began to throw planks and timbers into the churning water, hoping they would provide flotation for the floundering lifesavers. This only made things worse, for if any of the timbers or planks had struck the men, they might have died. Now the lifesavers had to dodge debris in the water. Somehow three lifesavers managed to get close enough to the pier to grab ropes thrown to them, and they scrambled out of the water. The other lifesavers reached the overturned surfboat and held onto it until they reached shallow water, where onlookers rushed out and pulled them to safety.

Taken to the Customs House, "the crew, now more dead than alive," donned dry clothing brought to them from their station. As the lifesavers began to revive, a man came rushing in to report *Johnson* breaking up on the beach. The crew hurried as fast they could to the station, where they found that Surfman Hatch had readied the beach apparatus gear. It was 11:30 P.M., two hours after *Johnson* had first been sighted, when the lifesaving crew set up the beach apparatus opposite the stranded barge. The wreck lay in about the same location of the wreck of *Sophia Minch*. At 11:55, the Lyle gun roared and Surfman Eveleigh, faithfully still at his station, grabbed the line. Within ten minutes, the crew of six men and one woman were safely ashore.

The lifesaving crew had braved freezing water for almost an hour with very little rest before taking off the sailors from *Johnson*. For days afterward, the bruised and chilled men limped about their duties.

Within eleven days the crew of the Cleveland U.S. Life-Saving Service Station managed, against great odds, to rescue a total of twenty-nine people from three ships. For this amazing feat, the entire crew won the Gold Life Saving Medal.

Surfman Frederick T. Hatch, who played a prominent role in all three rescues, left the U.S. Life-Saving Service and joined the U.S. Lighthouse Service in Cleveland. In 1891, Lighthouse Keeper Hatch further distinguished himself in another rescue, for which he received the Gold Bar attachment—for a second award—to the Gold Life Saving Medal. Frederick T. Hatch became the first person since the establishment of the award in 1876 to receive the Gold Bar for two major rescues.[18]

AN ABILITY TO IMPROVISE

Nine years after Keeper Charles Goodwin's efforts in Cleveland, the early morning beach patrol of the station at Hog Island, Virginia, on 23 February 1892, spotted a steamer's running lights too near the shore for safety. Quickly, the beach patrolman burned the flarelike device known as a Coston signal to warn off the ship. The steamer's navigation lights disappeared. Concluding he had warned off the ship, the patrolman continued his rounds. Upon arrival at the station at sunrise, the beach patrolman reported the incident to Keeper John E. Johnson. Keeper Johnson climbed to the lookout tower and surveyed the area. At this early morning hour, the weather was misty, with a northeast gale. Through the mist, Johnson spied the masts and stack of a steamer to the north of the station.[19]

Johnson quickly assembled his regular crew and one substitute, Joshua E. Barton. The nine lifesavers set out on a five-mile trek along the beach to the site of the wreck. What the Hog Island crew found was the 1,291-ton Spanish steamship *San Albano,* aground after missing the entrance to Chesapeake Bay, with twenty-seven sailors on board. The master had anchored, but the force of the sea caused the anchor to drag. Eventually, the ship struck shoals along the way, opening the seams of the hull and filling the ship with sea water. Finally, *San Albano* "grounded five hundred yards from the beach[,] a hopeless wreck."

Keeper Johnson and his crew found the ship lying broadside to the waves, with seas breaking entirely over it. Survivors aboard huddled by the deck houses. Slowly the seas shoved *San Albano* shoreward.

Johnson realized *San Albano* lay beyond the range of the Lyle gun. Even if the gun could manage to hurl the projectile to the stricken ship, the high seas and pounding surf made the use of the breeches buoy too dangerous and the surf car necessary. This meant another trip to the station. Keeper Johnson also ordered the surfboat hauled to the scene; he would have at his disposal all the tools for maritime rescue that the technology of the time offered.

The lifesavers took the station horse and made the long journey back to the unit. Another team of horses then brought the surf car to the wreck site. It was two o'clock in the afternoon by the time the lifesavers had set up their equipment. Keeper Johnson aimed the Lyle gun and pulled the firing lanyard. The first shot fell short. On the second try, the line fell upon the deck of the ship. In their eagerness to pull the shotline on board *San Albano,* however, the ship's crew allowed the line to chaff against the wreckage and it parted.

The rising tide and high surf drove the lifesavers back farther and farther from the water's edge, thus increasing the distance to the wreck. Finally, the wreck was out of range. With night fast approaching, Keeper Johnson decided to try the surf boat, "despite the gloomy assertions of experienced men in the crowd on the beach that no boat could live in the surf."

Dragging the boat up the beach to windward of the wreck, Johnson and his crew launched into the howling surf. The wind, sea and current, however, swept the lifesavers past the wreck. Johnson and the surfmen managed to work the boat to the beach and, with great difficulty, land it. Upon reaching safety, the life-savers emptied the water-filled surfboat. Undaunted, the crew pulled the boat farther up the beach and attempted yet another launch. Again, the seas and current proved too much, although the boat came closer to the wreck. The surfmen managed, again with great difficulty, to reach the beach a mile downwind from the ship.

Watching these futile efforts from on board *San Albano*, some of the crew, against the orders of their captain, managed to lower the only remaining lifeboat of the steam ship, and somehow seven sailors reached shore. In the official report of the wreck, the inves-tigating officer noted that this "circumstance [was] so exceptional under such conditions that it may be noted as little less than mirac-ulous." Sunset and darkness now made the rescue more difficult.

Keeper Johnson learned from the men who reached shore that the sailors on the ship were still safe and dry in the deck house, so he decided to rest his men. They had labored against the storm all day without food. A group of civilians volunteered to keep watch at the site while the crew tried to get some rest.

After a few hours of much needed rest, the lifesaving crew again rejoined their battle against the sea. The ship remained out of range of the Lyle gun. Keeper Johnson hit upon an idea. He had the Lyle gun lashed to the beach apparatus cart, with the shotline box tied to the forward axle of the boat cart. He put in an extra heavy charge of gunpowder. The lifesavers pushed the cart into the water as far as possible. Standing waist deep in the surf beside the cart, Keeper Johnson fired the Lyle gun. The plan worked. After the projectile landed just over the rail of the ship, the shipwrecked sailors, this time mindful of the chaffing, carefully worked the shotline toward them. The lifesavers and some onlookers now went on with their work to set up the beach apparatus. Soon the sailors aboard the wreck tied off the hawser.

It took eight trips to bring the nineteen officers and crew safely ashore. After interviewing the survivors, Keeper Johnson learned that one sailor from the ship, against orders, had tried to make it to the beach during the night on a plank and died. The district inspector of the U.S. Life-Saving Service who investigated the wreck wrote, "Great credit is due the keeper and crew of the Hog Island Station for their brave and persistent efforts, and every man did his whole duty."

The heroic efforts of many crews of the U.S. Life-Saving Service receive praise by those who understand the history of the service. Keeper John E. Johnson not only showed bravery but also exhibited another trait: the ability to improvise quickly in the face of danger. For the rescue of *San Albano,* Johnson received the Gold Life Saving Medal, and his surfmen all received the Silver Life Saving Medal. Later, the Spanish government awarded the entire lifesaving crew a medal of honor for their work.

2 | Unflinching Heroism

Until the second decade of the twentieth century, the best technology could do for wrecks beyond the range of the beach apparatus were rescue boats powered by human muscle. Oar-powered boats, both coastal lifeboats and surfboats, were the simplest of the major rescue equipment used by the U.S. Life-Saving Service, but they were also the most dangerous.

In 1873, Sumner I. Kimball obtained funds to purchase a 30-foot coastal lifeboat from England's Royal National Lifeboat Institute (RNLI). Coastal lifeboats are different from lifeboats used on board ships. English coastal lifeboats were heavy, weighing between seven hundred and one thousand pounds, and launched from land into the sea. These boats had air chambers in the bow and stern, and the early boats had a valve that would release the water in the upper part of the boat, thus making it self-bailing. All coastal lifeboats hereafter would remain self-righting and self-bailing, although the technology of how these traits were accomplished changed over the years. The boats also had sails for longer offshore work. After a period of testing, the English type of lifeboat became the heavy weather boat for certain locations in the service. On the East Coast of the United States, most stations had to drag a boat across a beach and launch directly from the beach. The great weight of the lifeboat made this nearly impossible. Eventually, the service stationed coastal lifeboats on the Great Lakes and the West Coast. Stations in these locations were usually close to the water and used an inclined marine railway to launch the boats. At first, the lifeboat met with resistance from the crews at stations. They were used to the lighter and easier-to-handle surfboats. Then an interesting thing happened. Observing the heavy weather these boats could survive, crews began to regard them as "something almost supernatural." The wooden lifeboat underwent modifications over the years, but in its basic design, it remained the mainstay for coastal lifeboats in the U.S. Life-Saving Service and U.S. Coast Guard until 1964.[1]

Surfboats were the boats most used by the U.S. Life-Saving Service. These craft were generally light, open, of shallow draft, and usually measured between twenty and twenty-seven feet in length. This was the most popular boat for fishermen on the eastern seaboard—the backbone of the service's crews on that coast. The lightness of the boat made it easy for small crews to handle, they were maneuverable, and they performed well in short pulls in heavy surf. All these attributes were important, as most East Coast stations had to drag their surfboats across a beach and launch them directly into the surf. Throughout the history of the service, there was no standardized surfboat, and a large variety of the craft served at the stations.[2]

Most of the rescues accomplished by the early boats of the U.S. Life-Saving Service were close to shore. Anyone who has had to row a large pulling boat in calm water knows how difficult it is to handle oars that are at least twelve feet long. Rowing in steep seas made this an operation for only the skilled.

A DAUNTING TASK

The *Ephraim Williams* of Providence, Rhode Island, bound from Savannah, Georgia, encountered a severe storm near Frying Pan Shoals, near Cape Hatteras, North Carolina, on 18 December 1885.

Mountainous seas battered the hapless barkentine for three days. By 21 December, it had drifted, with sails in shreds, dangerously close to the shoals, and the captain ordered the anchor dropped to stop its headway. The anchor would not hold, and *Ephraim Williams* began to drag ever closer to sure destruction. Crews of lifesavers at Durant's, Creed's Hill, Cape Hatteras, and Big Kinnakeet Stations had spotted the ship and followed it along the beach. Eventually, all the crews gathered at the Cape Hatteras Station, but "such a fearful surf was thundering in" and *Ephraim Williams* lay so far offshore that "it was absolutely impossible for them to do anything." The lifesavers remained at the Cape Hatteras Station awaiting the dawn to see if the barkentine would clear the shoals. First light revealed *Ephraim Williams* had somehow cleared the shoals and "fetched up" in surf that old-time surfmen declared was the "heaviest and most dangerous they had seen for years." The barkentine was stranded six or seven miles northeast of the Cape Hatteras Station and approximately five miles offshore from the Big Kinnakeet Station.[3]

The crew from Big Kinnakeet rushed back to their station. Exhausted from their long night's vigil, they ate a quick breakfast to restore their strength. Just as they were finishing, Keeper Benjamin B. Dailey of the Cape Hatteras Station arrived with his crew and the station's surfboat drawn on its carriage by horses. Keeper Patrick H. Etheridge of the Creed's Hill Station, substituting for an absent member of Dailey's crew, accompanied this group. It was 10:00 A.M., and the lifesavers saw no indication that anyone remained alive on board *Ephraim Williams*. Then a lifesaver spotted a distress flag fluttering from the ship. Crews from Cape Hatteras and Big Kinnakeet prepared for the seemingly impossible pull of at least five miles, one way, in mountainous seas.

Lashing down everything that might break loose in the boat, and despite a piercing wind, the crews took off any clothing that might impede them in case the boat capsized. The men then donned their cork lifejackets and shoved their boats into the waters of the inner bar. Keeper Dailey and his lifesavers were the first to move off into an "almost unbroken wall of tumultuous water."

Dailey's boat went over the breakers of the inner bar, which were "immense in themselves," then the surfboat's crew faced the full fury of the sea at the outer bar, half a mile farther out. Witnesses on the shore held out little hope for the boat to withstand the savage pounding. Dailey kept his boat on station while he waited for a "slach," a brief period when the seas slacken. The slach arrived. Dailey exhorted his crew to give way together. The boat shot across the bar. The Big Kinnakeet Station's crew arrived at the outer bar and waited for a slach. None arrived. "Very much against their inclination," the crew returned to the beach.

Meanwhile, Keeper Dailey's crew fought the high seas in their long pull to *Ephraim Williams*. The seas were so high that witnesses on the beach at times could see the entire interior of the boat. Onlookers felt the boat would surely pitch pole, that is, go end over end. The lifesavers struggled at their oars for over two hours. In our modern age, the effort expended by the seven-man crew is almost unimaginable. As the surfboat approached *Ephraim Williams,* Keeper Dailey faced the daunting task of transferring the nine sailors from the ship to the plunging and rolling small boat. The heavy seas prevented him from laying the boat alongside the ship's hull. Dailey dropped the boat's anchor off *Ephraim Williams'* quarter and shouted to the captain of the ship to pass a line to the surfboat. Playing out anchor line from the small boat while pulling the line from the ship, Dailey brought the boat close enough to take the sailors on board one at a time.

Once all the sailors were on board, Dailey weighed anchor and the crew pulled toward shore. With sixteen men in the boat, the surfboat was down to its gunwales. On the trip to the beach, Keeper Etheridge relieved Daily at the sweep oar so that he could rig a sea drogue to steady the boat. The high following seas swept the boat quickly to the beach, where both lifesavers and rescued sailors tumbled safely out onto the shore.

The service called the work of Keeper Dailey and his crew "one of the most daring rescues by the Life-Saving Service since its organization." Deservedly, the entire crew earned the Gold Life Saving Medal.

A SEETHING MASS OF BREAKERS

Almost two decades after the rescue of the crew of *Ephraim Williams,* another harrowing rescue took place off the shores of North Carolina. The three-masted schooner *Sarah D. J. Rawson,* with a crew of seven sailors and a cargo of lumber, departed Georgetown, South Carolina, bound for New York, on 2 February 1905. Five days later, the schooner worked heavily northward under short canvas in a gale, high seas, and thick fog. *Rawson* ran aground in the breakers on the south side of Lookout Shoals and became a total wreck.[4]

When the ship struck, the master shouted orders to take in sail. A heavy sea swept the decks while the sailors tried to carry out the orders of their captain. Jacob Hansen, a Norwegian seaman, was swept to his death into the surf, while the other sailors clung desperately to the ship. The wind and seas gradually pushed the schooner onto the shoal. Violent seas carried away its boat and fore and aft deck houses, shifted its cargo, and its spars began to fall. The crew scrambled as high as possible in the wreck. In a classic bit of understatement, the official report of the wreck noted that the sailors found "their situation gloomy and almost hopeless."

At the Cape Lookout U.S. Life-Saving Station, about nine miles north by west of the wreck, Keeper William H. Gaskill had a problem: nearly all of his surfmen were ill, suffering from an outbreak of influenza. Gaskill knew the weather could bring on a wreck in his area of operations. To help his sick surfmen, the keeper kept a sharp watch in the lookout tower. At 12:05 P.M., while scanning the sea with his binoculars, Gaskill "caught, through a rift in the fog, a glimpse of the schooner's topmost spars." Knowing the ship had grounded, he went down to call out his sick crew. In the words of the official investigation into the wreck, "Not one [surfman] shrank from what all knew must at best be a long and wearisome pull in wintry weather over 18 miles of rough sea."

The wind proved favorable, so the surfmen put up the sail, and the boat arrived off the wreck by 4:00 P.M. What greeted the lifesavers must have made even the most seasoned surfman hesitate and wonder about the work ahead of him. The schooner lay upon its starboard side, in a "seething mass of breakers." Its deck houses had been carried away, as well as most of the masts. Breakers tossed lumber and other wreckage, threatening the "safety of the lifeboat and the lives of its crew." Despite the severe damage to the schooner, six of the ship's crew remained alive.

Cautiously, Keeper Gaskill and his surfmen tried to work his boat alongside the wreck. Debris and breakers drove them back. They made six attempts without success. Later, the skipper of *Rawson* said that "he momentarily expected to see the lifeboat pitched end over end in the turbulent sea." The U.S. Life-Saving Service noted that "the cool and skillful management of the keeper and crew" kept the boat from sinking.

Darkness began to fall. Keeper Gaskill anchored his boat nearby, hoping "that in case of the schooner's going to pieces they still might be able to rescue some or all of the sailors." Throughout the long, cold night, the lifesavers had to fend off pieces of wreckage that threatened to hole their craft. During the night, the wind increased, and Gaskill moved his boat to a better location. From the stern of the boat, Gaskill kept up a barrage of encouragement to lift his surfmen's spirits and to make sure they did not drop off to sleep. With the hurling debris, sleep meant disaster. The crew remained at their stations without food or water throughout the night.

At dawn's light, the lifesaving crew again approached the hulk. The sea continued very high. Keeper Gaskill decided to await the turning of the tide, which would help improve conditions. At 11:00 A.M., the wind and sea moderated. The lifesavers, suffering from influenza and having spent twenty-four hours in a small open boat, again took to their oars. Gaskill maneuvered the craft to about fifty yards upwind from the wreck and anchored. He slowly let out the anchor line, and his surfmen steadied the boat, allowing it to drop between the breakers and debris. A surfman stood in the boat and threw a heaving line to the sailors on *Rawson*. On board the wreck, a sailor caught the line, quickly wrapped it about himself, and leaped into the sea. The lifesavers just as quickly pulled the seaman into the boat. Five more times the lifesavers pulled sailors to the boat, rescuing all survivors. In yet another humane act, the surfmen took off their own oilskin jackets and wrapped them about the sailors. They then turned to their oars.

The official report of the U.S. Life-Saving Service spoke of the "unflinching heroism" of the lifesaving crew. For their work on 9–10 February 1905, Keeper William H. Gaskill and his crew earned the Gold Life Saving Medal.

MUSCLES AND GASOLINE

By 1909, the U.S. Life-Saving Service had begun experimenting with the use of gasoline engines in boats. An unusual rescue off the coast of New Jersey in 1912 combined the age-old use of oars with this new technology. On the gale-swept morning of 30 December, the tug *Margaret,* with barges in tow, bound from New York to Norfolk, Virginia, struck a submerged object off the coast of New Jersey. The captain, recognizing the severe damage to the tug, ordered the barges cut loose. He maneuvered *Margaret* toward the beach, trying to ground it. The lookout watch at the Avalon Station spotted *Margaret* grounded in the breakers three hundred yards from shore.[5]

Keeper Frank Nichols of the Avalon Station knew that a boat from the Tathams Station, south of the wreck, had the advantage of the wind at their stern once clear of the surf zone. Nichols called the Tathams Station on the telephone and passed on the information about *Margaret.* He then rounded up his own crew and set out to help the lifesavers from Tathams. Keeper Harry McGinley of Tathams hauled his power surfboat down to the beach. Making an open beach launching is one of the more difficult feats of seamanship—doubly so in storm conditions. The boat's bow must meet the incoming surf squarely. A little off, and a breaker can swing the craft broadside and roll it back onto the beach, possibly injuring the crew.

When Keeper McGinley launched the power surfboat, he had the engine and propellers turning over to give the boat steerage way. The surf was so high, however, that the engine also needed the muscles of seven surfmen at the oars for the craft to make it past the first line of breakers. The boat filled with water during the transit. Fortunately, the surfboat was a self-bailer and the water drained away.

The wind and seas increased. Once beyond the breakers, however, the lifesavers had everything to their backs and soon neared *Margaret,* resting with its bow to the beach. Only the upper part of the pilothouse and three to four feet of the bow remained. Everything else, including *Margaret*'s boats, had been carried away.

As seas lashed the pilothouse, Keeper McGinley judged the situation. The least-exposed place on the wreck was the starboard bow. McGinley gave each lifesaver "a few quick-spoken instructions." The crew through hard effort kept the boat in one position the best they could in the heavy seas, waiting for McGinley's command to go at the right time. Seeing a chance, McGinley ordered full power on the engine. He maneuvered the boat so it rode the crest of a wave toward *Margaret.* Unfortunately, fifty yards from the tug, the wave died. To make matters worse, at just this moment, "two towering seas" raced at the small boat. McGinley ordered full astern to meet the waves head on, but the craft responded too slowly. The first wave broke over the heads of the surfmen and they completely disappeared from the view of *Margaret*'s crew. The boat and surfmen shook off the sea just as another wave struck and again drenched the lifesavers.

As the battle continued, seas, wind, and tide carried the lifesavers and their boat 250 yards away from the tug. Surfmen again took to the oars to help the engine. The boat gained some yardage, then lost it again to the sea. To keep from going over the side, the surfmen at times found it necessary to stop rowing and grab onto the boat's seats. This continued for more than half an hour. Finally, the lifesavers' efforts paid off: they came to within 25 yards of the tug.

Keeper McGinley later said that surf around the wreck "was the worse [sic] he had ever encountered in 29 years" on the New Jersey beaches. The master of *Margaret* reported that on two attempts to reach the tug, the lifesavers' "boat was flung so high above the surface of the water" that he could see light underneath its entire length. The gale increased. It now "attained almost the velocity of a hurricane and the seas became miniature mountains." Despite getting so close, the weather and current kept the surfboat from reaching *Margaret.*

By this time the lifesavers were at the end of their endurance. A breaking wave capsized the surfboat. Five of the crew, including Keeper McGinley, reached the upside-down boat. But three surfmen came up so far away that, after futilely trying to reach the surfboat, two struck out for the shore.

While McGinley clung to a blade of the propeller, four of the surfmen held onto the bilge strips of the boat that were now in the air. Several times the men tried to right the boat, but without success. Eventually, all managed to reach the safety of shallow water. Bystanders and the Avalon Station crew carried the exhausted and shivering lifesavers to a roaring fire in an abandoned barn.

By 2:00 P.M. the wind had slackened and shifted to the west, further knocking down the surf. Keeper Frank Nichols of the Avalon Station felt that he could now try to make an attempt. He sent his crew for his surfboat, which arrived at 3:30 P.M. As the Avalon surfboat made ready for launching, an unusual problem arose. The Tathams crew, even after their beating from the sea, wanted a place in the rescue boat. Both keepers worked out a solution. The two keepers and three surfmen from each station made up the rescue crew that pushed out to *Margaret.* This surfboat depended solely on the muscles of the crew.

The combined crews launched into the surf and bent to their oars. Almost immediately, the seas swept the surfboat past *Margaret.* The surfmen continued struggling at their oars. They reached close enough to see "the haggard faces of 10 despairing men" in the pilothouse as waves broke over the top of them. The wreck now afforded no sheltered area for the lifesavers to make their approach. What little remained of *Margaret* stood a good chance of breaking up.

With more favorable weather, the lifesavers approached the tug. As the surfboat "shot in under the tug's bow," a surfman heaved a line to the pilothouse and a sailor on board the tug secured the line. The line between *Margaret* and the surfboat came taut. At just this time, the surfboat swung broadside to a series of waves, filling the surfboat with frigid water and carrying away five oars. The two keepers struggled with the steering oar and worked the boat around to a better position. They managed to get close to the tug, and *Margaret*'s crew quickly clambered into the surfboat.

Just as the last man got off, "a giant comber lifted the boat high in the air and sent her smashing against the side of the tug, staving in three of her planks." Despite this damage, the surfmen shoved off with only three oars. The weight of eighteen men in the surfboat lowered the boat almost to its gunwales. Somehow, despite this, the lifesavers managed to reach the safety of the beach.

For their successful rescue, the U.S. Life-Saving Service awarded the Gold Life Saving Medal to the lifesavers who made one or two trips into the storm.

3 | Prodigies of Heroism

When Sumner I. Kimball reorganized the U.S. Life-Saving Service, one of his first actions was to place stations closer together. He decreed that there be no more than five miles between them. Surfmen patrolled between the stations, ensuring a lookout along the shoreline. Usually, a surfman's patrol took him about halfway to the next station. At the halfway point, he met the surfman from the next station and the men exchanged metal tags proving they had completed their rounds. As the service grew, stations were set farther apart. A surfman carried a watchman's clock with him, and he walked until he reached a key at a designated location. At the location, the patrolman inserted the key into the clock to prove completion of the patrol. Every night, and during thick weather, surfmen donned oilskins, picked up metal tags, or watchman's clock, and Coston signals and slogged off on their patrols. The Coston signals burned like flares and were used to either warn off ships approaching too close to the beach or to let a wrecked ship know help was nearby.

The idea of a walk along a moonlit beach might seem like pleasant, or even romantic, duty. Try the same beach in a November gale in New Jersey or along Lake Superior in the winter. Many contemporary accounts of beach patrols speak of the shoreline as "clad with ice" and little more than "pathless deserts in the night." At times, surfmen plodded their way "through the soft sand, in spite of flooding tides, bewildering snowfalls, overwhelming winds, and bitter cold."[1]

During daylight hours, surfmen kept watch from lookout towers either built into the station or set a short distance from the unit. Beach patrols and lookout watches were low technology, but they worked. The 1899 annual report of the service, for example, recorded that 143 ships veered away from danger by patrolmen lighting Coston signals.[2] Many dramatic rescues began with a beach patrolman running back to his station to give the alarm.

UNTIL THE BLOOD RAN

At 1:30 A.M., on 25 November 1888, *Oliver Dyer* anchored just inside the entrance to the Portsmouth, New Hampshire, harbor. The schooner, out of Saco, Maine, was returning to its home port laden with coal and shipped a crew of five. It became the third ship riding at anchor near the entrance.[3]

Earlier in the evening, the winds increased. Heavy surf crashed upon the beach. As thermometers registered temperatures below freezing, it began to snow. Keeper Silas H. Harding, in charge of Jerry's Point Station, scanned the three ships at anchor near the entrance to the harbor.[4] Harding had a surfman place a heaving stick and line near a patrol box on the beach; this proved to be a prophetic move.

At 5:45 A.M., on 26 November, Surfman Ernest Robinson, trudging along the north beach patrol, saw *Oliver Dyer* dragging its anchors. He fired off a Coston signal to let the ship's captain know help was on the way. Robinson ran back to the station to inform the keeper. Keeper Harding called out all hands and, while the crew assembled, ran to the shore. There, he observed the ship brought up by its anchors just outside the surf zone, about four hundred yards from the station. Keeper Harding's first thought was to launch the station's boat. Just as the lifesavers started to ram the boat into the pounding surf, he observed the schooner's head fall off to the south and the vessel again running before the gale. The keeper realized the schooner's chains had parted. Just as quickly, he knew that the hapless *Oliver Dyer* would strike about 150 feet offshore upon the ragged ledges east of the station. This new set of circumstances caused Harding to change his tactics. He now knew the breeches buoy offered the best way to reach the sailors on the schooner. Station crewmen stopped the launch of the boat and instead brought the apparatus from the boathouse to the scene.

As Keeper Harding had foreseen, *Oliver Dyer* slammed into the ledges. *Dyer*'s crew took to the rigging to escape the pounding sea. Quickly, lifesavers set up the breeches buoy apparatus. A large wave caught the schooner broadside and threw it thirty or forty feet inshore. *Oliver Dyer* crashed onto the rocks. Raging seas boarded the ship, pushing *Oliver Dyer* farther into the rocks. Frigid seas made complete breeches over the ship, plucking one sailor from the main rigging some forty feet above the main deck. Harding later reported that "when the first seas went over the vessel there was nothing of her in sight but her top masts and lower mastheads, and it [was] a miracle that every soul was not washed into the sea."

Harding realized the shipwrecked crew in the rigging would never be able to handle the shotline and other lines needed to effect a rescue by the breeches buoy. As Harding took all this in, *Oliver Dyer,* pushed by the strong seas, came to rest within fifty to seventy-five feet of a large, flat rock. Harding ran to the patrol box where he had earlier stowed the heaving stick and line and ran back to his lifesavers. Keeper and surfmen then timed the seas and pushed out to the large rock. A sailor from the schooner jumped into the churning seas. Disregarding his own safety, Surfman Ephraim S. Hall dived into the frigid water to help the sailor. Just as Hall and his shipmates were helping the sailor to the rock, a huge wave swept the lifesavers and sailor into the tempest. Fortunately, everyone was swept into the water on the lee side of the rock. Had they fallen seaward, undertows might have swept them to their deaths. Even so, the lifesavers took a beating. Sharp rocks severely cut their hands "until the blood ran," but they managed to regain the relative safety of the large flat rock.

While the lifesavers struggled to regain the rock, the ship's cook jumped over the side. Surfman George W. Randall immediately plunged into the frigid, heaving water after the man and grabbed him before the undertow took him out to sea. The lifesaving crew had safely landed two of *Oliver Dyer*'s crew. Two more remained aboard the schooner.

Keeper Harding took the heaving stick and line and threw it to the men on the ship. Harding gestured for the sailors aboard *Dyer* to use the heaving line to haul aboard a stouter line. After getting the line on board the ship, Harding signaled that the sailors should fasten the line under their arms and leap into the sea. Harding's lifesavers would then pull them ashore. The plan worked.

Harding, making sure he had rescued everyone, sent Surfmen Randall and Winslow A. Amazeen to the rock to see if they could spot the man washed from the rigging. The two made their way to their precarious perch. No sooner had they reached the rock than a huge sea swept them into the water. Amazeen caught Randall and, as the sea rolled back, they clung desperately to the rock. Both managed to reach safety.

Lt. Charles F. Shoemaker, the U.S. Revenue Cutter Service officer who investigated the wreck and rescue of *Oliver Dyer*, wrote, "It is not often that life saving crews are called upon to perform service under such circumstances as environed this case, but this crew was equal to the emergency, and under the able leadership of Keeper Harding performed prodigies of heroism seldom equaled. Every man in this crew came within an ace of losing his life, from the keeper down; so that while they were doing their utmost to save the crew of the wreck, they were in turn saving the lives of each other . . . Every time they went to that sea-combed rock upon their errand of mercy it was a forlorn hope, but they . . . [met] it and conquered."

For their abilities to conquer the elements on this night and save four of the five man crew of *Oliver Dyer,* Keeper Silas H. Harding and his lifesavers earned the Gold Life Saving Medal.

AN OLD HAND AT HIS BUSINESS

Almost eight months later, and many miles to the south of where Keeper Silas H. Harding and his crew struggled to rescue the crew of *Oliver Dyer,* Surfman Rasmus Midgett of the Gull Shoal Station, North Carolina, did not rush back to his station when he found the wrecked *Priscilla.* The keeper's log entry for 18 August 1899, states, "R. S. Midgett, surfman No. 1 on south patrol from 3 A.M. to sunrise. He found a wreck broken to pieces 3 miles south of the station and on stern was ten men. He managed to save them all without coming to station to report."[5]

The story begins on the night of 17 August when the 643-ton barkentine *Priscilla,* bound from Baltimore to Rio de Janeiro, ran afoul of the infamous weather off Cape Hatteras. Fourteen people were on board, including Capt. Benjamin E. Springsteen, his wife, their twelve-year-old son, and an older son who was the first mate. Winds were more than one hundred miles an hour, according to Captain Springsteen, "blowing a hurricane from the northeast, and the seas were running mountain high." After 9:00 P.M. the crew felt *Priscilla* touch bottom lightly. The seas smashed through the cabin skylights and quickly drenched everyone below deck. Twenty minutes later, the ship again grounded, this time violently and permanently. Captain Springsteen ordered the third and second mates forward to cut away the port rigging. No sooner had this been done than the masts carried away.

There was still hope, for no lives had been lost. The captain now ordered all hands on deck as the seas began breaking over the hull "with irresistible fury." Suddenly, as the captain clutched his youngest son in his arms, a huge wave slammed into the ship, tearing the boy from his arms and sweeping his wife, his other son, and the cabin boy overboard to their deaths. In that split second Captain Springsteen lost his entire family. Fifteen or twenty minutes later, the hull split in two. The crew managed to remain on the afterdeck section, calling vainly and desperately for help.

Rasmus Midgett, making the south patrol on horseback from Gull Shoal Station, came riding along the beach and spotted boxes, barrels, and other debris coming ashore. The surf on the beach was so high that it reached the saddle girth of his horse, but the evidence of a wreck urged him on. Peering through the darkness, he spurred his horse along for another two miles then reined up and listened. A sound drifted in the darkness, then another. He had found the wreck. But what could he do? If he rode back to the station, it would take hours to return with help. The ship's crew would surely be dead by the time assistance arrived. Midgett hesitated only long enough to think things through. He then dismounted and waited, timing the waves as they pounded in and then receded. Having gauged them, he ran into the ocean after the receding waves, coming as close to the hulk as he dared, and shouted for the sailors to "jump overboard, one at a time, as the surf ran back, and that he would take care of them." He then ran back before the rushing surf.

To the crew of *Priscilla*, it must have seemed an insane plan, but what other hope was there? Midgett watched the surf then screamed for the first sailor to jump. Over the side the sailor went. Rasmus rushed forward, grabbed the man, and dragged him to shore. Seven times he escaped with his rescued sailors. Now another dilemma confronted the surfman. Three sailors, including Captain Springsteen, were unable to move.

Hesitating only a minute, Surfman Midgett plunged into the water again, fought his way through the pounding waves to the side of the hulk, seized one of the lines, and pulled himself hand over hand to the deck. "Panting for breath from his . . . exertions," he lay there for a few minutes, trying to catch his breath and rest his aching muscles. Regaining his strength, Midgett put one of the helpless sailors over his shoulder, slid down the rope into the sea, and fought his way through the flaying surf to shore. Twice more Midgett made his harrowing trips. Captain Springsteen proved extremely difficult, as he weighed at least two hundred pounds. As

Midgett struggled up the beach under this burden, a wave "dashed over them." Midgett dug his toes in and fought to keep upright. He later admitted that he thought his "time had come." Finally, all ten surviving crewmen of *Priscilla* lay panting and shivering on the beach. Midgett headed the seven who could walk toward the station. He gave his coat to Captain Springsteen, who had suffered the most serious injuries, and set out to get help. Eventually, all were warming themselves at the station.

Lt. C. E. Johnson, U.S. Revenue Cutter Service, following regulations, investigated the wreck and rescue. His report stated that Midgett "doesn't deserve any special mention" for the rescue of the first seven sailors, as the men, to some degree, were able to help themselves. Johnson admitted it "was a hazardous piece of work," but, he noted, Midgett "was an old hand at his business." The rescue of the remaining three crewmen, however, was "quite a different matter." Surfman Rasmus Midgett received the Gold Life Saving Medal.

NO MEN COULD HAVE DONE MORE

Four years after Ramus Midgett's amazing feat, at about 4:00 P.M. on 20 January 1903, the twenty-seven-year-old barkentine *Abiel Abbott,* bound to New York from Turks Island, West Indies, approached the Barnegat, New Jersey, light. Capt. Israel B. Hawkins set his ship's course based upon this supposition. The master had unfortunately misidentified the lighthouse, and four hours later *Abbott* grounded. Captain Hawkins quickly had his crew furl the sails while he sent up distress signals. Almost "instantly" a red Coston signal came from the beach patrolman, Surfman Barton P. Pharo of Ship Bottom Station, New Jersey. Pharo hurried the mile and a half to his station and informed Keeper Isaac W. Truex of the wreck. Keeper Truex turned out his crew. Before departing the station with the beach apparatus, Truex telephoned the station to the north, Harvey Cedars, and the unit to the south, Long Beach, for assistance. Truex and his six surfmen then departed for the wreck site.[6]

Meanwhile, the weather began to worsen. *Abbott* had grounded broadside to the seas. By the time the Ship Bottom Station crew arrived at the wreck site, the wind and seas had driven the ship heavily onto the bar and waves were breaking over *Abbott*'s deck. Lifesavers from the Ship Bottom Station quickly set up the Lyle gun and apparatus and Keeper Truex fired the first projectile to the barkentine, which fell short. The lifesavers retrieved the projectile, while Truex selected a heavier shotline and measured a heavier charge of black powder. Truex again yanked the firing lanyard. The official report on the wreck describes what happened next: "The shipwrecked sailors failed to find [the projectile] for the reason that it fell amidships or forward, and as they were confined to the extreme after part of the vessel they could make no search except in their immediate vicinity. The whole hull, except the quarter-deck, was by this time submerged, and the constantly increasing waves were rolling deeply over it."

Through the darkness and spray, Keeper Truex saw only "a glimmer of a scarcely perceptible light." Nevertheless, he fired another shot, and the projectile landed on board the ship. Again, no one on board gathered in the shotline. Yet again the keeper fired and successfully placed another projectile on board the wreck. For some unknown reason, the sailors on board the *Abbott* did not begin securing the lines. At just about this time, the crews from the other two stations arrived on scene. The gale raged at full force and the night remained pitch black. In the words of the official report of the wreck, "No sane man would try to launch a boat before daylight." If the "old hulk would only hold together until daylight," the sailors on board *Abbott* might still make it ashore safely. Throughout the long hours of the night, the barkentine heaved and strained "with ominous signs of breaking up."

Between three and four o'clock in the morning, the mainmast fell. It hung by the stays to the other two masts until around five in the morning. Then the lifesavers on the beach heard the noise of all the masts going. This was more than one sailor on board *Abbott* could take. He panicked and leaped over the side to his death. Eight other sailors were still alive under the mizzen mast when it went, and they fell into the churning sea. Five more sailors managed to hold onto the mast and work their way up it to the hulk and clung to the top of the cabin; the rest perished.

At first light, the lifesavers launched their boat. Besides the high seas, they faced great danger from the broken planks and timbers of *Abbott* churning in the waves. Two keepers, Truex and George Mathis of the Long Beach Station, manned the sweep oar. Six surfmen of the Ship Bottom Station, and two additional surfmen from Long Beach, pulled at the oars. The remaining lifesavers took their places in the water. A surfman stood on each side of the boat, holding it and trying to clear the debris, waiting for the right moment to launch. "The men in the water," reads the official report, "were compelled to exercise the utmost skill and nimbleness to escape the flying debris and none were hurt seriously, although several were bruised."

When an opportunity came to launch, "the surfboat instantly shot out." The lifesavers on the beach did not think their fellow lifesavers stood a chance with the debris in the heavy seas. By this time there were many bystanders on the beach. One, Henry S. Jones, said to the investigating officer, "When the boat was launched I thought the chances were ninety-nine in a hundred that it would be smashed. It was a most dangerous time, and I certainly expected to see the lifeboat destroyed."

The lifesavers in the surfboat pulled to the location of *Abbott*. Spars, masts, timbers, and other dangerous debris formed a barrier around the barkentine "impossible to penetrate." Lt. Ellsworth P. Bertholf of the U.S. Revenue Cutter Service, the investigating officer, wrote, "The life-savers exerted every effort of strength and skill at their command, but finally had to give up and return to the beach, well worn-out and their boat battered and scarred."[7] Hapless sailors still clung to the top of the cabin.

Just as the surfboat arrived at the beach, the sea tore loose the top of the cabin, which began to move with the other debris toward the shore. Immediately, the lifesavers again launched the surfboat. With the cabin top moving within the debris field, the lifesavers managed to pluck off four sailors. The fifth, thrown into the sea, clung to a hatch cover, but the lifesavers also managed to recover this sailor. Of the five sailors brought from the sea, one died soon after reaching safety.

Lieutenant Bertholf later wrote, "Nothing that could be done was left undone by the life-saving crews, and the loss of life in this wreck was due to circumstances beyond the control of men. The launching of the surfboat twice through the heavy breakers, filled with timbers and all sorts of wreckage, bristling with nails and spikes and bolts, was a feat that the Ship Bottom crew and the Life-Saving Service have reason to be proud of."

The captain of *Abbott* remarked, "I do not see how the life-savers launched the boat at all . . . Finally, when the cabin top broke adrift, they launched their boat again when no man could have expected it. I did not think it possible for them to get to us, but somehow they did . . . I think it is a miracle that I am alive to tell this tale. No men could have done more than the life-savers did."

For their work at the wreck of *Abiel Abbott,* the service awarded Gold Life Saving Medals to the entire crew of the Ship Bottom Station. In addition, Keeper George Mathis and Surfmen M. D. Kelly and W. E. Pharo of the Long Beach Station received Gold Life Saving Medals for their work in the rescue.

4 | Angels in Oilskins

Very little is known about the people who served in the U.S. Life-Saving Service (an anonymity shared by those serving in the modern-day U.S. Coast Guard). Unlike many government services, the U.S. Life-Saving Service was a local affair. People living near the stations looked upon the units as belonging to them, not some far-off organization in Washington, D.C. The service was national, but so many men served their local stations that this perception grew. Too, crewmen became a part of the community. They helped in everything from fighting fires in nearby homes to helping free horse and buggies mired in beach sands.

Service headquarters gave the man in charge of a station the title "keeper," but crewmen, locals, and newspapers addressed him as "captain." A keeper had to be at least twenty-one but no more than fifty-five years of age. (There was one exception to this regulation: the enlistment of Joshua James, detailed in chapter 5.) He also had to have a "knowledge of notation, numeration, and the four elementary rules of arithmetic." The keeper had to be an expert in the "management of the surf-boats and of the use of the various apparatus used in the service." Keepers were responsible for all aspects of running the station, including selecting and managing the crew. Two other important duties were to keep a journal, or log, of the station's activities and to file wreck reports. Keepers exerted as much control over the station as did the captain of a ship.[1]

Known as "surfmen"—the title comes from the fishermen along the East Coast who launched their boats into the surf from the beach—crewmembers were "able bodied and experienced." They had to be "under forty-five . . . able to read and write," and they had to "possess a thorough knowledge of surf boats."[2]

The service employed crews only part time, when wrecks were most likely to occur. Known as the "active season," on the East Coast this varied by location but usually stretched from November to April. Surfmen signed on for a season and, if they performed to the keeper's satisfaction, returned the next season. Only the keeper remained at a station year round. As the service expanded to include the Gulf of Mexico states, the Great Lakes, and portions of the West Coast, the active season changed gradually. Along the West Coast, stations remained open all year.

The size of a station's crew was small and depended on the number of oars needed to row the largest boat assigned to the station (one man per oar). At surfboat stations, generally located along the East Coast, this would be six surfmen and the keeper. At lifeboat stations, usually located along the West Coast and on the Great Lakes, there were eight surfmen. Near the beginning of the twentieth century, another man was added to the units to help in the winter season.

By the 1880s, surfmen were wearing uniforms. On the left sleeve of the uniform jacket, each lifesaver wore a number that indicated his position in the crew. Surfman Number 1 was the most senior and the second in command.

Today, very few Americans recognize the name of the U.S. Life-Saving Service. The men who served in the organization have largely slipped behind the veil of history. Most who served did not write about their experiences, so there are few letters and diaries that later generations can study.[3] Only a few individuals have managed to garner publicity, and they must represent all who have served.

Most keepers in the U.S. Life-Saving Service possessed a reputation for leadership, and one of the best examples of such leadership was keeper Lawrence Oscar Lawson of the station at Evanston, Illinois. Lawson was born on 11 September 1842 in Kalmar, Sweden. He first went to sea at the age of eighteen, and after he emigrated to New York in 1861, he continued his profession of sailor.[4]

By 1864, Lawson had made his way to Chicago, where he worked as a fisherman and sailed on lake ships. Five years later, he took up residence in Evanston, Illinois, just north of Chicago. Next, he journeyed across Lake Michigan to Ludington, Michigan, but he returned to Evanston in 1878. With the establishment of a station at Evanston, Lawson's vast experience at sea made him a natural for the position of keeper. He received the appointment in 1880 and remained in this position for close to twenty-three years. In 1902, a local newspaper commented that Lawson, at the age of sixty, was still able to undertake the "daily boat drill and manipulates the heavy beach apparatus." By the next year, 1903, however, failing vision caused his "retirement." Members of the U.S. Life-Saving Service did not have a retirement system as we know it today. If a keeper or surfman could not pass a physical, he left the service with no retirement money. At best, keepers and surfmen were granted a one-year compensation for injury in the line of duty.

Newspapers recorded that Lawson was responsible for "the rescue of over 500 persons from the stormy waters of Lake Michigan." He died on 29 October 1912. Although he served honorably for years, Keeper Lawson's career was not far different from that of many other long-service keepers. What makes Lawson different is the makeup of his crew.

In 1871, Northwestern University received the gift of a lifeboat, and in 1876, a red-brick station followed. Selected students of the university crewed the boat. "At the annual graduation exercises, the life-saving boat was handed down by the seniors to the junior class and a new captain was chosen." Eventually, the U.S. Life-Saving Service felt the unit needed a seasoned mariner to "make seamen of the eager but inexperienced students." Lawson, with his years of sea experience, received the call.

One can only imagine how an old salt felt about whipping a group of young college students into shape to survive the dangers of maritime rescue. There were concerns that an outsider "would not be able to get the cooperation of the student crew," and that "the appointment of Captain Lawson would be the first step toward the severance of relations between the university and the life-saving station." Keeper Lawson surprised everyone. Within a short time, his skills "succeeded in winning the loyalty of the crew." Former crewman George H. Tomlinson recalled that "the most eventful period of the station's history began with the appointment of Captain Lawson . . . as keeper of the station. He . . . won the love and respect of all who entered the university in that time. As a member of one of the student crews who served under him, I can attest to his courage, ability and fineness of character—a rare soul such as does not often come into one's life."

Tomlinson remembered, "No one who has not had the privilege of waking [Lawson] in the middle of the night to report some emergency could envision him coming out of his bedroom into the hall with his long white nightgown and his long graying beard, with one hand searching his ribs, either for the answer or to help him awaken, and the other hand twisting his beard back and forth."

Lawson apparently never lost his patience, even when things were a little different at Evanston. In 1900, for example, the *Chicago Tribune* reported that Lawson feared his surfmen were not keeping their minds strictly on their duties because "every afternoon, before and after drill, the members are surrounded by bevies of fair maids, and in the evening the lake shore is dotted with groups of young women talking to the lifesavers. Even when it is time for their favorites to go on patrol duty the young women do not depart, but turn their attention to the reserve men."[5] Many years later, one of Keeper Lawson's sons would relate that in the "summer, when the boys wore white suits, we got quite a few calls from people around Calvary cemetery. They thought they were seeing ghosts."

William E. McClennan, another former member of the Evanston crew, remarked that Lawson never gave up hope "so long as human lives were in danger." The proof of this statement came on Thanksgiving Day 1889.

The fifteen-hundred-ton steamer *Calumet* ran into one of Lake Michigan's late fall storms. Earlier, the ship had struck a submerged object in the Detroit River and had sprung a leak, and the steam pumps keeping the ship afloat failed. The leak, combined with the storm, spelled the end of the ship. To save his crew of seventeen, the captain ran his vessel aground. Then he ordered the hold of the vessel flooded to prevent the ship from going to pieces in the pounding waves.[6]

Calumet grounded at 10:30 P.M., and some time passed before a local resident discovered the wreck and wired the Evanston Station, about twelve miles away. Keeper Lawson received the telegram shortly after midnight and immediately checked with the local railroad station. A freight train to transport his boat and beach cart would not be available until 7:30 A.M., but Lawson learned a passenger train might stop to carry his crew to the site. Lawson next ran through the snow to a livery stable. He rented teams of horses to pull the boat, beach equipment, and some of the crew by road. Then, Lawson and the remainder of the crew went by train to survey the situation and be ready to act when the teams arrived.

Meanwhile, *Calumet* lay submerged almost to its main deck, waves breaking over it. Overlooking the wreck site were seventy- to eighty-foot brush-covered bluffs. Once the horse-drawn beach apparatus arrived, at 7:00 A.M., Keeper Lawson had it rigged. After two unsuccessful shots, he realized that the wreck lay well beyond the six-hundred-yard range of the lines. Lawson's last recourse was the boat, despite the heavy surf that lashed at the foot of the bluff. Aided by fifty soldiers from nearby Fort Sheridan, and some civilians, the lifesavers cut brush and wrestled the boat down the bluff to the beach.

Working waist-deep in the icy water, the soldiers and civilians managed to get the boat into position, windward of the wreck and facing lakeward. As the next wave lifted the boat, they gave a mighty push. The lifesavers sprang to their oars. Near the bluff, an immense breaker struck the boat as it crossed the inner bar. Lawson almost went overboard from his position at the stern sweep oar. Before he could recover himself, a second wave dashed over the boat and filled it to the boat's seats. Lawson ordered a surfman to ply the bailing bucket, while the other lifesavers strained at their oars. The strong current drove the boat far to the leeward, giving them a long and hard pull directly into the gale.

Lawson stood in the stern, facing the full brunt of the storm and exhorting his crew. Freezing temperature encased the crew's clothing, oars, and oarlocks with sheets of ice. A former crewman on the rescue later recalled, "I really believed we were all going to our death. Still I knew the captain and I knew the other boys. . . . I never knew exactly how we reached the steamer, but I will never forget the welcome those poor devils of sailors gave us. We took a half dozen of them on board the boat, and then set out on our return trip. I thought the following waves would swamp us, but as each cloud of spray went by I could see the Captain standing at his post, his long beard matted with ice, but his voice as calm as if we were on drill."

Soldiers and civilians on the beach rushed the survivors to a blazing bonfire and gave them hot coffee. Lawson again ordered his crew out into the gale. "The second trip was like the first, except that it was harder, for we were cold and worn out, but we made it to safety," recalled the former lifesaver. "When the time came for the third trip, some of the boys felt mighty like giving up, and the soldiers and the bystanders told us we had done enough. Still, we went without a murmur when the Captain ordered us out, and somehow we got through safely." All eighteen sailors on *Calumet* came safely ashore.

By the time the lifesavers reached the beach on their last trip, they were in terrible shape, so numb they could scarcely walk. For their outstanding rescue on this cold, stormy night in November, the entire crew of the Evanston Station received the Gold Life Saving Medal. The service rarely awarded an entire crew the Gold Life Saving Medal. From 1878 to 1908, the service presented entire crews with the medal only ten times. Keeper Lawson's student crew of 1889 is one of these select ten. Former crewman William E. McClennan said it best: "Without [Keeper Lawson] as a leader through almost a quarter of a century, the Evanston life-saving crew could hardly have won for itself much more than average fame."

If information on keepers is sparse, the background of the surfmen is almost nonexistent. Men in the service signed articles of agreement for a stipulated period, and the only information on them comes from the sparse data entered on the personnel rolls and the few references found in keepers' letters. The myth of the surfman closely parallels that of the keeper: a waterman with many years of experience who spent a great deal of time at one station, advanced slowly, and eventually was promoted to keeper. One surfman will serve as a representative for all the forgotten men who filled the ranks of the service.

Theodore Roberge was born in Crookston, Minnesota, in 1889, the youngest of thirteen children.[7] His father was a police officer in St. Paul. Part of the Roberge family moved to Seattle, Washington, where Theodore entered the U.S. Navy as an enlisted man at the age of sixteen. He served for one enlistment on the Yangtze River Patrol in China, then returned to Seattle to work as a tinsmith. After serving as a coxswain for one enlistment in the U.S. Revenue Cutter Service, Roberge entered the U.S. Life-Saving Service in 1911. Roberge's first duty station was at Cape Disappointment, Washington. This unit, on the north side of the Columbia River, has an operational area in some of the highest surf in the United States. Within two years of entering the service, he had received a Gold Life Saving Medal, along with his fellow lifesavers from the station at Cape Disappointment, for his work at the wrecking of the tanker *Rosecrans* on deadly Peacock Spit near the mouth of the Columbia River on 7 January 1913. Roberge remained in the service and advanced to lieutenant in the U.S. Coast Guard before his retirement in 1941.[8]

In 1902, John W. Dalton published a book titled *The Life Savers of Cape Cod* in which he listed all the keepers and surfmen serving on Cape Cod, as well as short biographical entries for each. This is the only known book that gives a glimpse of the surfmen near the end of the U.S. Life-Saving Service era. One station, Cahoon's Hollow, will serve as an example of the crews of the service.[9]

The average age of the six surfmen at Cahoon's Hollow in 1902 was just over thirty-eight, with the oldest, at fifty-six, Surfman Number 1 Freeman W. Atwood, and the youngest, at twenty-five, Surfman Number 4 Stanley M. Fisher. The crew averaged just over nine years of service, with Surfman Atwood claiming twenty-five years. The average was lowered because three of the surfmen had only one year of service each. Five of the surfmen were married and had children; Surfman Number 3 Edward Lombard and his wife Nellie Howes Lombard had four boys. All but one of the six came from the Cape Cod area.

Surfman Fisher's background was particularly interesting, although he was the youngest man on the crew and the surfman with the shortest time in the service. Born in 1877 in Nantucket, Massachusetts, Fisher began his working life as a boatman and fisherman. Like many of his time, he headed west. Arriving in Texas, he worked "on a stock ranch." But "tiring of this kind of life," he enlisted in Company K, Sixth Regiment, U.S. Army. He saw combat in the Philippine Islands, including "six hot battles and several minor engagements." At the end of his enlistment, he returned to Cape Cod. Upon his return, Fisher became "a member of a volunteer crew which rescued a crew from a sunken vessel in Vineyard Haven Harbor during the gale of November, 1898, receiving gold and silver medals as a recognition of his bravery."

Surfman Number 6, Clarence L. Burch, the junior man in the crew, also led an adventurous life. Born in Provincetown, Massachusetts, in 1875, Burch first worked as a boatman and fisherman. In addition, he sailed in coastal ships. Succumbing to the lure of gold, Burch, "along with a party of prospectors," spent "a short time" in the "Klondike gold region." Apparently none the richer, Burch returned to his native Cape Cod and entered the U.S. Life-Saving Service in December 1902. He was married to Dorothy McKenzie and they had two daughters.

FEMALE LIFESAVERS

Most of the rescues from U.S. Life-Saving Service stations were by men, but there are interesting exceptions. At most stations, only the keeper's family could live on a unit. In many isolated units, married surfmen had to construct buildings for their wives and children just outside the boundary of the station. When everyone departed the station after the active season, the keeper and his family looked after the station. During this inactive period, it was not unusual for the keeper's family to help with rescues. On the Gulf of Mexico, for example, the Norwegian bark *Catharine* grounded during a hurricane on 7 August 1894. The "breakers ran so high" that the beach apparatus, the most complicated equipment used by the service, was used. Two of the keeper's daughters, Sara Louise and Visa Broadbent, helped rescue the entire crew of *Catharine*. For their work, they received a gold medal from the king of Sweden.[10]

Another interesting story is that of Edith Morgan of Hamlin, Michigan. On 23 March 1878, before the opening of the active season, a strong northerly gale struck northern Lake Michigan.[11] The bitterly cold wind quickly whipped up pounding waves. A small boat carrying two men capsized. Both men clung desperately to the boat. The nearest U.S. Life-Saving Service station was Grand Point au Sable, where Keeper Sanford W. Morgan held sway. The only people available to help the two men were Keeper Morgan, his two sons, one of whom was a boy, and his daughter, Edith. Morgan realized his family could not row the surfboat in such a storm, so he opted to use a small fishboat. He put his son at the sweep oar to steer the small boat, while he, Edith, and his other son pulled at the oars. To reach the capsized boat, the family of lifesavers would have to cross two bars, over which the waves were breaking heavily. The official U.S. Life-Saving Service's report notes that Edith "did her part" in the hard work which followed, but with such a small craft, the boat barely made it over the first bar, and by the time the would-be rescuers had reached the second bar, the boat "was nearly swamped." Keeper Morgan decided to put about. Upon reaching the beach, he immediately dispatched his older son, James, to town to gather a volunteer crew and return with the surfboat. Meanwhile, father and daughter began to clear a path for the surfboat "through a great mass of logs and driftwood" that covered the beach. Edith and her father worked "with such energy" that when the crew arrived there was a clear path for the launching of the boat. Edith helped in ramming the surfboat into the waves, and eventually the two stranded men came safely ashore. Just before Christmas 1879, Edith again proved her courage.

On 21 December, *The City of Toledo,* a steamer, grounded two hundred to three hundred yards offshore in a gale-whipped snowstorm. The ship swung and lay broached in ten feet of water, seas breaking over it. In this bitterly cold weather, the waters sweeping over *Toledo* quickly froze, and soon the ship "resembled an iceberg." The steamer struck between the U.S. Life-Saving Service stations at Grand Point au Sable and Ludington. The keeper of the Ludington Station set out with volunteers and the surfboat.

Rescuers faced high banks of ice rafted upon the beach. After finally getting the boat into the water, the cold weather caused the thole pins (used to keep the oar in place while rowing) to clog with ice, preventing the use of oars. Keeper Morgan had assembled some volunteers and started to the wreck site with the beach apparatus. Edith was among the volunteers.

Once this group arrived, the Lyle gun shot the messenger line and the volunteers rigged the heavy hawser between ship and shore. The severe cold, however, continued to hamper the rescue effort. Ice clogged the tackle and lines, making the process painfully slow. Edith, along with the other volunteers, stood in the piercing wind, in fifteen inches of snow for five or six hours working the apparatus. Keeper Morgan decided to set out in the surfboat, and he successfully brought some passengers from *The City of Toledo* ashore. For her heroic work on these two occasions, Edith Morgan received the Silver Life Saving Medal, the first woman to do so.

UNDAUNTED COURAGE

The single feature that leaps out about those who served in the U.S. Life-Saving Service is their indomitable courage. From somewhere deep within them, they found the strength to make perilous rescues in life-and-death situations. Indeed, some rescues almost defy belief. Take, for example, the rescue headed by Keeper W. W. Griesser of the station at Buffalo, New York.

At 2:20 P.M. on 21 November 1900, with winds whipping across the harbor at eighty miles per hour, two large scows were torn loose from their moorings. Trapped on board the scows were several men. The lookout tower watch at the U.S. Life-Saving station sounded the alarm, and Keeper W. W. Griesser and his crew leaped into their lifeboat. They managed to have a tug tow them to a point three-quarters of mile windward from the drifting scows.[12]

Keeper Griesser brought the lifeboat to just outside the surf-line, then ordered the anchor set. Griesser planned to play out the anchor line slowly and work the boat to the scows. The anchor began to drag. As the small lifeboat entered the surf, some breaking waves completely buried it. Suddenly, an extremely large wave parted the anchor line and the craft pitchpoled, that is, it went end over end. All but one of the lifesaving crew catapulted into the cold, churning surf. Griesser and his lifesavers made the tough, numbing swim of at least a quarter of a mile to the beach. Recovering on the beach, the lifesavers learned a man on board one of the scows had fallen over the side and was in desperate shape. A quarter of a mile separated them from the sailor in the water. Luckily, a locomotive engineer, who happened to be nearby, said he would transport the lifesavers on his train.

Arriving at the location, Keeper Griesser spotted the unfortunate man desperately clinging to some slippery piles some four to five hundred feet from the beach, "the seas constantly breaking over him." The seas were so high that "at times . . . he was completely out of sight." Griesser knew the use of the boat was impracticable. If help did not reach the man quickly, he would surely drown. Griesser decided he would swim a line out to the man and called on another surfman to accompany him. As the two lifesavers were about to again enter the frigid, treacherous seas, onlookers warned them they did not stand a chance of coming back alive.

Keeper Griesser's reply: "Wait until we try, he can not make it to us; we will try to go to him."

Griesser looped one end of a line around his arm and he and his surfman dived into the lake. The breakers threw both men back upon the beach. Again they tried to reach the man. They swam about fifty yards from the beach, but a large wave threw the surfman swimming with Griesser against an old pile, injuring him, and then swept the injured lifesaver toward the beach. Bystanders on the beach helped the surfman ashore.

Keeper Griesser continued swimming alone for fifteen long minutes, until he managed to reach a pile sixty to seventy yards from the beach. There, he managed to hold on, trying to gain his wind and strength. Griesser then pushed off, renewing his solitary battle with the strength of the furious lake. In the words of the official report on the rescue, Griesser was "many times beaten back from 100 to 200 feet," yet he never gave up. When a large breaker came toward him, the keeper dived beneath it. During the battle, a large floating telephone pole passed over the lifesaver, considerably injuring him, but he never gave up.

Finally, Griesser approached close enough to throw the line to the man, telling him to make it about his waist and then to cast off from the pile. The battered victim had only enough strength to put the line around his wrist. Before the unfortunate man could push away, a large wave hit the pile and tangled the line in the pilings.

The same sea flung Keeper Griesser at least a hundred feet from the pilings. For the first time since entering into combat with the lake, the lifesaver would later recall, a "fear entered" his mind that he "might fail." Even the official record catches something of what spurred Griesser onward: "The imperiled man was begging piteously . . . to save him and crying out that he could hold on but a few moments longer."

Undaunted, Griesser first battled to regain the lost one hundred feet. Successful, he next had to swim in the churning water among the piles to free the line. After an exhausting fifteen minutes, Griesser gave the man the signal that the line was free and he should shove off. Griesser watched as those on the beach pulled the man ashore and then the keeper struck out on his own for shore. The exhausted Griesser reached shallow water and needed help the remaining distance to the beach.

Keeper W. W. Griesser's successful swimming battle against the power of the lake "consumed three-quarters of an hour." Even the U.S. Life-Saving Service found his efforts almost too harrowing to believe, except "for indisputable evidence of that you performed the marvelous feat, which was, indeed, effected only at the extreme peril of your life."

The official report of the U.S. Life-Saving Service captures Keeper W. W. Griesser's heroic and lonely efforts over a century ago: "Physically weaker men could not have endured the strain, while men less brave although of equal strength would long before have given up." For his Herculean efforts, Griesser rightfully received the U.S. Life-Saving Service's highest award for valor: the Gold Life Saving Medal.

AT THE OARS FOR SIXTY MILES

Two years after Keeper Griesser's heroic actions, and east of the Buffalo Station, the crew of the station in Charlotte, New York, again proved the determination of the crews of the service. Eleven days before Christmas 1902, the train master of the New York Central Railroad at Charlotte received a telegram to notify Keeper George N. Gray of the Charlotte Station that a farmer living near Lakeside had reported a vessel "showing signals of distress." Strong winds, high seas, and snow swept Lake Ontario, while thermometer readings plunged. Keeper Gray realized that Lakeside, located about twenty-three miles to the east, would be an almost impossible pull against heavy seas. The harbor being frozen over, Gray requested from the New York Central Railroad a special car to reach Lakeside. The lifesavers fought deep snow to get their boat to the depot. Before departing, Keeper Gray telegraphed Lakeside to have teams of horses waiting for them.[13]

What the farmer had spotted was *John R. Noyes,* which had departed Charlotte three days earlier under the tow of the steamer

John E. Hall, bound for Deseronto, Canada. The two ships ran into fierce weather on Lake Ontario. At 8:00 A.M. on 13 December, *Hall* became disabled and the captain made the decision to cut *Noyes* loose. Meanwhile, the lifesavers and their surfboat arrived near Lakeside in the midst of heavy snow and high winds. Weather conditions required horse-drawn sleds. Snow drifts of at least six feet blocked the road, and the crew helped shovel a passage through many drifts. The lifesavers did not reach the launch site until 11:30 P.M.

Undeterred, they donned their cork lifejackets and prepared to shove off into the churning lake. Before launching, Keeper Gray arranged with local townspeople to have a roaring bonfire going on the beach. Gray then gave the order for the boat to shove off. The extremely cold weather caused fog to rise from the lake. The lifesavers pulled for approximately seven miles through the thick vapor. Gray, using his compass, kept searching in the murk, at intervals burning Coston signals. After about three and a half hours, Gray ordered the boat back to the beach. The crew then camped by the roaring fire.

Only a few hours later, at first light, Keeper Gray put into action his plan for the day. He ordered a surfman to the top of a nearby windmill to scan the lake. While the surfman kept watch, Gray and the remaining crew would launch the boat. If the surfman up the windmill spotted the wreck, he was to signal the boat which way to go. Before Keeper Gray could launch, the surfman yelled that he saw something in the far distance. With a pair of binoculars, the surfman could see *Noyes.*

Keeper Gray took a bearing off his compass and again launched into the lake. At first the surfboat had the wind to its stern and the lifesavers had few problems for at least ten miles. This ended when the wind shifted and came off the beam of the boat and the waves picked up, making a dangerous passage in the trough. Spray passed over the boat, freezing to the surface of the craft and coating the lifesavers in ice. Keeper Gray and his crew fought these conditions for yet another ten miles. When the lifesavers arrived off *Noyes* at 11:30 A.M., they found the schooner "drifting helplessly, sails blown away, anchors gone, cabin stove in, leaking badly and heavily coated with ice. Its crew, consisting of master, mate, two seamen, and a female cook, were suffering much from fifty hours' exposure, thirty-six of which had been without food. Some were hysterical, and had bidden one another good-bye, with the expectation of sinking at any moment." Making things even more difficult, the wind had picked up and the seas were "running high." Keeper Gray wrapped the woman in his "overcoat and provided her with mittens." Quickly, the lifesavers managed to place the survivors safely into the surfboat and pushed off for the beach.

The return to safety was no easier than the long pull to the schooner; the surfboat had to remain in the trough of the waves, which constantly threatened to swamp the heavily ladened small craft. At 4:30 P.M., after spending almost the entire daylight hours rowing on the frigid, storm-tossed lake, the lifesavers approached the beach about a mile and a half from their launching site. Keeper Gray and his crew could not rest, however. The large accumulation of ice on the boat prevented the lifesavers from landing the survivors. They "were compelled to carry the rescued people ashore, through the water and ice, on their shoulders." Once the rescued people were ashore, the lifesavers rowed to a spot further down the beach where horses could drag their boat ashore. Keeper Gray then arranged for his crew, the rescued sailors and his boat to return to Charlotte by rail.

Keeper Gray would later learn that *Noyes* stranded and went to pieces on the Canadian shore. If not for heroic work against seemingly overwhelming odds, the ship's crew would have gone the way of the steamer that originally towed them: *John E. Hall* went down with the loss of all hands.

The official report of the rescue noted the lifesavers were "under oars from 11:30 P.M. of the 14th to 4:30 P.M. of the 15th continuously, with the exception of about two hours, having pulled in a heavy seaway nearly or quite 60 miles, and all were more or less frostbitten, some seriously." Although there is no official record of the longest distance covered by lifesavers of the U.S. Life-Saving

Service, the distance rowed by the crew of the Charlotte Station to rescue the sailors of *Noyes* must rank at the top.

The rescue of the crew of *John R. Noyes* is one of the best illustrations of the dedication and bravery of those who served in the U.S. Life-Saving Service. Surfmen did everything from riding a train and shoveling snow to climbing a windmill and rowing for many hours to save lives on Lake Ontario. For their work on this cold December night in 1902, Keeper George N. Gray and his crew deservedly received the Gold Life Saving Medal.

5 | March 1902

The "sea has no generosity," wrote sailor and writer Joseph Conrad. Two incidents in Massachusetts in March 1902, incidents that sent shockwaves throughout the U.S. Life-Saving Service, prove Conrad's simple but eloquent observation.[1]

On Tuesday night, 11 March 1902, the tug *Sweepstakes* approached Boston towing the coal-filled schooner barges *Wadena* and *John C. Fitzpatrick*. The captain of the tug stared through the windshield of the bridge at an infamous New England nor'easter. A prudent mariner, the captain sought shelter, but the tug ran aground in Shovelful Shoal, off the southern end of Monomoy Island, Cape Cod.

Alerted to the grounding, the crew of the Monomoy U.S. Life-Saving Service Station pulled out to the barges and tried to refloat them. This effort proved unsuccessful. The weather showed no sign of improving, so the lifesavers took each of the five-man crews off *Wadena* and *John C. Fitzpatrick* to their station. Everyone arrived safely ashore at 3:00 P.M.

Sweepstakes remained by the barges for a few days but finally left the scene for repairs as the tug *Peter Smith* took over the vigil. The owners of the barges hired workers to remove the cargos and refloat both schooner barges. The weather was intermittently foul, and the work continued between lulls. On Sunday, 16 March, the weather took a turn for the worse. *Peter Smith* maneuvered around *Wadena* and removed all but five of the barge's workers.

At 8:00 the next morning, the beach patrolman on the south patrol from the Monomoy Station reported to Keeper Marshall N. Eldridge that the barges seemed safe. A few minutes later, however, the telephone rang at the U.S. Life-Saving Station. The captain of *Peter Smith,* moored at Hyannis, Massachusetts, asked Keeper Eldridge "whether everything was all right with the men on board *Wadena.*"[2]

Keeper Eldridge decided to check on the condition of *Wadena* for himself. He made his way to a point some three miles from the station for a better view. Rain lashed the area, lowering visibility, and strong southeast winds whipped up the seas. Added to this, the ebbing tide cut across the wind-driven water, "making a very ugly sea." Eldridge's viewpoint was about half a mile south of the point. Keeper Eldridge at first saw nothing out of the ordinary. During a short break in the weather, however, the keeper caught sight of a distress signal, "a summons he could not disregard." He hurried to a telephone in the south watchhouse and called Surfman Number 1, Seth L. Ellis, the station's second in command. Eldridge briefed Ellis of the distress and ordered him to get the lifesaving crew into the boat and get moving. The lifesavers quickly donned foul-weather gear, entered their boat, and pulled hard to Eldridge's location.

Keeper Eldridge clambered on board and took the sweep oar. He advised his surfmen that he intended to go out to *Wadena.* His crew put their backs into their oars while Eldridge guided the boat through heavy seas. During the trip to the barge, the boat shipped "perhaps a barrel of water." Near noon, Eldridge brought the small boat under the lee of the barge, just abaft the foremast, with his bow pointing toward the stern of *Wadena.* Someone from the barge heaved a line to the lifesaving boat, and Eldridge secured his boat to the barge. He ordered the five men on board *Wadena* to scramble twelve to thirteen feet down a rope from the barge into the pitching boat.

The owner of the barge, Capt. C. D. Olsen of Boston, a rather large man, lost his grip about halfway down the line and fell into the boat. He landed "with such force" that it broke the second thwart in the boat, putting the lifesavers sitting on that seat at a "great disadvantage" in the coming pull to safety.

Keeper Eldridge ordered a surfman to cut the line connecting the boat to the barge and to shove off. Eldridge tried to maneuver the boat through the breakers around the stern of *Wadena*. "While the surfmen holding the port oars were backing hard and those on the starboard side were pulling," a sea struck the boat, "pouring a great deal of water into it." Panic struck the five men from the barge. They stood up and grabbed the surfmen, crowding them out of their places on the thwarts. This "practically made anything like effective work impossible." Amid this panic, a larger wave struck the small boat, capsizing it into the cold, heaving sea. The lifesavers, and those from the barge, tried to cling to the boat. "Twice the life-savers righted it, but each time the seas upset it." The frigid water began to take its toll. The five workers from *Wadena* were the first to succumb. Surfmen Osborne Chase, Valentine D. Nickerson, and Edgar C. Small soon slipped beneath the sea. Within minutes after this, Surfmen Elijah Kendrick and Isaac T. Foy also perished.[3]

Only Keeper Eldridge, Ellis, and Surfman Arthur Rogers remained. A larger wave knocked them away from the boat. Ellis and Rogers managed to regain the overturned boat, but Eldridge could not; he grasped a floating spar and drifted away to his death. Rogers cried out to Ellis to help him obtain a better grip. Ellis could not help him but yelled that they were drifting toward shore, to hang on and they would make it. Rogers weakly said, "I have to go," and slipped beneath the sea.

Ellis, still clinging to the overturned boat, slipped off his foul weather gear and boots and waited to see where the sea carried him. The overturned craft passed by the stranded *John C. Fitzpatrick*. The visibility was so low that those on board *Fitzpatrick* could not see *Wadena*. In his weakened state, Ellis thought he saw someone throw something into the water from *Fitzpatrick*.

On board *Fitzpatrick,* Capt. Elmer F. Mayo of Chatham, Massachusetts, in charge of the wrecking operations, saw what looked like a capsized boat drifting by, with someone clinging to it. Mayo remembered that earlier, through a momentary break in the weather, he had glimpsed a distress signal from *Wadena.* He quickly realized that the boat belonged to the U.S. Life-Saving Service. Mayo grabbed a large wooden fender and threw it over the side, hoping it would drift to the boat. It did not.

"Mayo now astonished his shipmates" with his decision to save whoever was hanging onto the overturned boat using only the barge's 12-foot dory. The dory had no equipment, having capsized the day before—not even oars or thole pins to hold the oars. Mayo disregarded these obstacles. His shipmates fashioned thole pins made of two pieces of "pine wood, a serving stick, and an old rasp were quickly driven" into the dory. Crewmen further improvised by sawing off two oars to fit the dory. With this, Mayo proposed to put out into the tempest.

"Mayo threw off his boots and oil jacket," strapped on a life-jacket, and leaped into the dory, which had been lowered to the side of *Fitzpatrick.* With "consummate skill," he maneuvered this jury-rigged dory alongside Ellis. The weakened Ellis managed to drag himself on board the dory. Mayo now had to bring Ellis to safety. His jury-rigged oars prevented him from returning to *Fitzpatrick,* and he could not pull for sheltered water. He had to attempt an open beach landing in high seas, the most difficult of beach landings, in his puny dory and with only two old sawed-off oars.

As he approached the beach, Captain Mayo judged the waves. At the last moment he saw someone on shore rushing out to help him. Surfman Walter C. Bloomer, who had remained on the beach to help when the Life-Saving Service boat returned, now "rushed into the surf to help Mayo beach" his frail dory.[4] The surfman helped Mayo and all three men returned safely to the beach.

For his heroism, Capt. Elmer F. Mayo received the Gold Life Saving Medal, as did Surfman Number 1 Seth L. Ellis. The service also promoted Ellis to the keepership of the Monomoy Station. In the history of the U.S. Life-Saving Service and U.S. Coast Guard, there have been only two incidents when seven crewmen were lost while on rescue from a shore-based station.

THE MOST FAMOUS LIFESAVER IN THE WORLD

The news of the loss of the Monomoy crew spread throughout the service. North of Monomoy, a legendary waterman received the news with sadness and determination that this would not happen to his crew. Two days after the Monomoy deaths, Keeper Joshua James of the Point Allerton Station took his crew out for additional boat drills. The boat launched into a heavy northeast wind, with the seventy-five-year-old keeper at the sweep oar.

Joshua James defies the anonymity typical of the personnel of the U.S. Life-Saving Service. Sumner I. Kimball, general superintendent of the U.S. Life-Saving Service, wrote that James reached the status of the "best-known lifesaver in the world."[5] He is a legend in Massachusetts and within the U.S. Coast Guard. Like most legends, it is sometimes difficult to keep fiction from creeping into the story of his life.

James began his legend as a lifesaver in December 1841, thirty-seven years before the official founding of the U.S. Life-Saving Service and one month after he turned fifteen. Born on 22 November 1826 in Hull, Massachusetts, the ninth of twelve children, he sprang from a maritime family. His father, William, owned a fleet of twelve ships. His mother, Esther Dill, earned a reputation for caring for others. Legend says that a traumatic event concerning his mother is probably the factor that led to Joshua's fame. On 3 April 1837, at the age of ten, Joshua watched helplessly as the schooner *Hepzibah* capsized, taking with it his mother and baby sister. "After that," according to family tradition, Joshua "seemed to be scanning the sea in quest of imperiled lives."[6]

Joshua followed in his father's footsteps and became owner of a ship, but at the age of fifteen he joined the Massachusetts Humane Society and worked as a volunteer lifesaver. Within a few short years, his reputation as a maritime lifesaver grew. A fire destroyed the records of the Massachusetts Humane Society in

1872, so all the documentation that survives about his service in the Humane Society is from secondary sources and family tradition. These sources show that Joshua participated in a number of rescues in violent weather. The society does have documentation of a bronze medal he received from the society for the rescue of the crew of the French brig *L'Essat* on 1 April 1880. The record also shows he received a certificate for work at the wreck of the *Delaware* on 2 March 1857. By 1876, the society had appointed James keeper of a number of their lifeboats and a "mortar" (a line-throwing device, similar to the Lyle gun) station. In 1886, James received a silver medal from the society for "brave and faithful service of more than 40 years." Three years later, he received a gold medal from the society and a Gold Life Saving Medal from the U.S. Life-Saving Service. Shortly after receiving these medals, James became the keeper of the newly established U.S. Life-Saving Service station near Hull.

Service regulations stated that keepers could be no older than forty-five years of age at the time of their appointment. Such was James's reputation, however, that Kimball, known as a stickler for enforcing regulations, granted Joshua's appointment at the age of sixty-two. Kimball later noted that this was the only age exemption in the history of the service. It was, he declared, "amply justified by his magnificent record during the subsequent . . . years of his service."[7]

Despite earning the title of the "best-known lifesaver in the world," James has yet to be the subject of an in-depth biography. Any such book would no doubt include the events that took place on 25–26 November 1888, when a severe storm swept into Massachusetts.

The nor'easter brought with it a blizzard. High seas, combined with a high tide, lashed the shoreline. The blizzard passed, followed by driving sleet and rain. Joshua James, feeling sure there would be work for him, made his way to the top of a hill, along with two volunteer surfmen, and surveyed the area.

Through breaks in the storm, a number of small schooners swung by their anchor chains. James knew no anchor or chain made would hold these ships, so he sent one of the accompanying surfmen to call out the volunteers. At two in the afternoon, James called out the volunteer beach patrol. The volunteers had no sooner started their difficult trudging through the storm than they located a three-masted schooner, *Cox and Green,* in trouble. The lifesavers drug the beach apparatus and lifeboat from the Massachusetts Humane Society's Stoney Beach Station half a mile away to the wreck site.

James loaded, aimed, and fired the line-throwing mortar, and soon the rope bridge stretched to the schooner. With precision, James's lifesavers brought the men ashore until all nine members of the ship's crew reached safety. Darkness now fell upon the beach, and seeing no other vessels in distress, the volunteers retrieved and stowed their gear. Before they could depart for their station, however, someone saw another schooner, *Gertrude Abbott,* slamming onto the rocks about an eighth of a mile farther up the beach. Again the volunteers slogged along the dark, storm-lashed beach. They discovered that the schooner lay out of range of the line-throwing mortar. The fury of the seas made any boat rescue attempt seem "suicidal."[8] James warned his volunteers that anyone pulling out to *Gertrude Abbott* in the boat might never return. He wanted only volunteers for this rescue. Despite this warning, "every man volunteered."[9]

Word of the wreck reached the nearby town, and the citizens arrived on the scene. They immediately built a large bonfire to light up the area. This also let the sailors on the schooner know that help was nearby.

James and his crew launched into the surf. The boat filled with water to the thwarts. The sea flung the boat back to the beach. James had the lifeboat emptied and again his crew launched into the violent seas. "Several times" they attempted the launch, and eventually, human muscle and James's skill at the sweep oar managed to work the boat out of the surf zone.[10] Still battling heavy seas, James maneuvered the lifeboat to the schooner's bow. A surfman heaved a line to the wrecked ship and a crewman on board the ship made it fast. Timing their jumps with the heaving boat, eight sailors, one at a time, leaped into the boat.[11]

James and his crew now faced great danger in returning through the raging surf in a heavily laden boat. Added to this danger were the jagged rocks in the area. The boat started toward the shore but struck a rock and nearly capsized about two hundred yards from the beach. A crewman catapulted into the churning sea, but James's well-trained crew managed to get him back into the boat. James shouted above the noise of sea and storm to remain with the boat as long as possible. The lifeboat again struck rocks, and in the turmoil oars were lost. This made maneuvering the boat even more difficult. A very large wave took the lifeboat, hurled it like a matchbox onto the beach, and broke into splinters. Miraculously, everyone escaped injury.

James and his surfmen were now soaked and dazed. Although James knew his men were worn out, and it was nine o'clock at night, he ordered the beach patrol continued. The decision was fortunate, for at three o'clock in the morning, a third ship came ashore. The three-masted schooner *Bertha F. Walker* grounded in the breakers about half a mile northwest of where *Gertrude Abbott* struck. Like *Abbott, Walker* lay out of the range of the line-throwing mortar.

The lifeboat lay in splinters upon the beach near *Gertrude Abbott*. Strawberry Hill, the next volunteer station, was four miles away. Horses and other volunteers drug the boat from that station to the new wreck site. This boat was unknown to Joshua James's crew. Although the crewmen were "skeptical" about the boat, they willingly pushed out into the raging sea, with James at the sweep oar. After "a bitter struggle," the lifesavers brought seven of the schooner's nine sailors safely ashore. Tragically, before the volunteer lifesavers came upon the scene, the captain and mate were lost when washed overboard.[12]

Even as James's crew worked to bring the survivors of *Bertha F. Walker* ashore, a man on horseback rode up and shouted there were two more ships in distress at Atlantic Hill, five miles away. The Hull lifesavers had been at it all night and the seemingly tireless crew had brought twenty-four sailors safely ashore.

Exhausted, bruised, soaked, cold and hungry, the lifesavers quietly readied their gear for the five-mile journey down the dark beach. Joshua James sent a message to the officer in charge of the Massachusetts Humane Society's station at Crescent Beach and Keeper George Brown at the U.S. Life-Saving Service station at North Scituate requesting additional help.

The Crescent Beach crew arrived at the scene first and found the schooner *H. C. Higginson* lying between two ledges of rock, decks awash. Anderson fired the line-throwing mortar, but the shotline parted. At just about this time, Keeper Brown arrived on scene and his surfmen quickly set up the Lyle gun. Just to reach the wreck site, Brown's crew had pulled their heavy beach apparatus through nine miles of snow and deep melting snow and ice in the face of the gale.

Both crews now fired their line-throwing devices, and both lines reached the schooner. But another frustration set in: both crews had their lines fouled. Almost as if scripted by Hollywood, James and his crew arrived at just this moment after pulling their boat through the "deep mud and slush" on the beach.[13] James took in the scene. He noticed a partly sheltered location, and without a word, the crew headed for it, launching off into the high surf. "After a heartbreaking struggle of forty-five minutes, the Hull life-savers had to yield to the storm gods and return to the beach."[14] The new boat came ashore stove in at two places.

The lifesavers searched around that dark beach for repair materials and, somehow, managed to patch the two large holes in the boat. Incredibly, they again launched their boat into the tempest. "After a fearful trip" during which the boat almost pitchpoled, the volunteers approached the schooner and saw that the survivors were barely able to move after spending fourteen freezing hours lashed in the rigging. The Hull crew had "a terrible time" unlashing the sailors and freeing them from their deathlike grips on the rigging. A large crowd on the beach formed a human chain stretching out a distance into the water to help the lifesavers land their boat.[15]

The fifth wreck that night, the *Mattie E. Eaton*, stranded high and dry and did not need the assistance of the lifesavers. The Hull lifesavers then "secured food" before beginning their long journey back to Hull. Still, their work was not yet finished. On the way home, the Hull crew came upon the sixth wreck, that of the abandoned brigantine *Alice*. After parting its moorings in Gloucester, the ship ended up grounded across the bay. Two men had boarded the ship and were marooned when their boat broke away. The weary Hull crew went to *Alice* and brought the two men ashore. This finally ended the long night's work.

In twenty-four hours, under fearful conditions, Joshua James and his crew had rescued twenty-nine seamen. James had led each rescue. Four of his crewmen had also worked on all the cases, and twenty others had worked at one or more of the ships. Both the Massachusetts Humane Society and the U.S. Life-Saving Service rightfully awarded their Gold Medals to Joshua James and his Hull crew.

Shortly after this terrible night, Joshua James became the keeper of the Point Allerton U.S. Life-Saving Station. While at this unit, eighty-six vessels wrecked in the area of operations under James's command. Sixteen sailors lost their lives in these wrecks, most during another terrible night, 26–27 November 1898.[16]

In July 1901, at nearly seventy-five years of age, James took, as required by service regulations, a physical. The seemingly tireless waterman passed successfully. Less than a year later, after the loss of the Monomoy crew, James took his crew out to drill in a strong northeast gale, working his surfmen for over an hour. Satisfied with the drill, he leaned into the sweep oar and maneuvered the boat to the beach near the station. The boat grounded on the beach. James leaped from his boat "as nimbly as a young man" and, after alighting, looked at the sea and said, "The tide is ebbing." After uttering this comment, Joshua James dropped dead upon the beach.

Perhaps the best epitaph for the old lifesaver is one he wrote after the storm of 26–27 November 1898: "We succeeded in getting every man that was alive at the time we started for him, and we started at the earliest moment in every case."[17]

PART II
1915–1964

6 | New Weapons against the Sea

As the twentieth century began, Sumner Increase Kimball, who had guided the U.S. Life-Saving Service for more than twenty-four years, could look back proudly on his accomplishments. He had molded the service into a well-known and well-received organization. In the National Archives, among the many scrap-books containing thousands of articles featuring the service, only a small number find any fault with the lifesavers. Kimball did have disappointments—the organization had no retirement system and no compensation for those injured in the line of duty, and crews received low pay—but he had good reason to be proud of the service. Very few government organizations, even today, have a reputation for being so well run, thrifty, and humanitarian. On 15 January 1915, the U.S. Life-Saving Service ceased to exist, and by 1940, few in the United States had ever heard of the organization. How did this happen?

Improved marine technology helped spell the end of the service. Its operating procedures dated from the 1870s, and rescue equipment consisted of either oar-powered small boats or beach apparatus gear. Rescues usually involved commercial vessels. Masters of early ships had few reliable aids to navigation and depended upon landmarks to guide them. In 1852, for example, there were only 333 lighthouses in the United States. Ships of the period were of wood and powered by the wind. Under these circumstances, most of the work of the service lay close to the beach. An unwritten premise of the service was that a crew would handle only one wreck per day or night. On the few occasions that premise proved inaccurate, the records of the service prove the crews could barely manage. Usually, volunteers helped save the day.[1]

By the beginning of the twentieth century, technology had changed almost all of the service's operating premises. Aids to navigation improved and increased. By 1913, the number of lighthouses had increased to 1,462, with electricity slowly taking over the type of illuminate used in the lights. Ships were, for the most part, steel- and steam-powered. The improved aids to navigation and ship construction now meant that vessels could safely stay farther off shore and were less likely to run aground.[2]

These maritime technological improvements helped mariners but added to the dangers of the U.S. Life-Saving Service. Launching an oar-powered boat from the beach into high surf for ships stranded near the shore was always a risky proposition. Usually, however, the danger lasted only a brief, though very intense and often harrowing, period. Now, with ships sailing farther offshore, the danger and time in rowing to a distress in storm-tossed seas increased.

The U.S. Life-Saving Service's 1909 annual report noted that "a new element in navigation . . . has in a remarkable degree increased . . . duties and notably added to the annual statistical showing. This new feature is the gasoline motor boat."[3] In other words, recreational boating had increased. Not only were there more boats in coastal waters, but often these craft were piloted by people with very little nautical experience, thus increasing the number of cases reported by the stations. Yet crews remained small and still used oar-powered boats. Further stretching the available resources was the fact that whereas crews previously had time to pull a boat on a cart along the beach to a site and launch, the increase in recreational boating cases made this very difficult. The service began to experiment with gasoline-powered lifeboats in 1910, and new boats appeared, but it was too little too late. (More on motor lifeboats later.)

The inroads of technology played an important role in ending the U.S. Life-Saving Service, but the treatment of the crews proved just as important. Lifesavers continued to work for low pay and no benefits. Contained within the records of the service are many examples of keepers and surfmen performing heroic rescues and serving honorably for more that twenty years. Long service in a hostile environment took its toll. When these old salts failed their physical examinations, they found themselves discharged from the service with no compensation. Some people, however, feeling they were contributing to some worthwhile effort, or failing to find other employment, continued to work for inadequate pay. Low salaries were not as important as the lack of a retirement system. A lack of retirements also held up promotions. Capt. Robert F. Bennett, a retired U.S. Coast Guard officer and a student of the U.S. Life-Saving Service, has graphically pointed out the result: by 1915 there were "keepers in their seventies manning the customary sweep oar while the strokes were manned by men in their sixties."[4] Clearly, maritime rescue demands stamina and agility. (Kimball had, of course, also aged. By 1900 he was sixty-six, and still there was no move to replace him as general superintendent.) Kimball tried but failed to correct these personnel problems. Given more time, he may have succeeded. In the end, however, it was politics that delivered the coup de grâce to the U.S. Life-Saving Service.

During the nineteenth century, the Progressive movement grew in political power. Progressives were drawn from both of the main political parties and sought to control what they saw as the excesses of a rapidly changing society. They championed social reforms, such as shorter work hours, child labor laws, and woman's suffrage. They also pushed to democratize the government and make the legislature more responsive to the people.

President William Howard Taft, under the acts of 25 June 1910 and 2 March 1911, appointed a commission to find ways to improve the economy and efficiency of the federal government.

Frederick A. Cleveland, an economist and financial adviser to the president, headed what became known as the Taft commission. The various small maritime police and safety forces of the federal government came under close examination. At the time, these forces were the U.S. Revenue Cutter Service, the U.S. Lighthouse Service, the U.S. Steamboat Inspection Service, and, of course, the U.S. Life-Saving Service, all of which, except for the Steamboat Inspection Service, were within the Treasury Department (Steamboat Inspection was within the Department of Commerce).[5]

The commission felt these organizations had served their purpose. They should end or become one organization. Under the proposal, the U.S. Life-Saving Service would come into the U.S. Lighthouse Service. No one has yet to completely describe the machinations that took place in the nation's capital, but in the end, the U.S. Revenue Cutter Service and the U.S. Life-Saving Service merged and became the U.S. Coast Guard. In 1939, in yet another movement to streamline the federal government, the U.S. Lighthouse Service came into the U.S. Coast Guard. During World War II, as a wartime measure, the Steamboat Inspection Service, now called the Bureau of Marine Navigation, came temporarily into the U.S. Coast Guard. The move was made permanent in 1946.

Lifesavers immediately reaped a benefit from the combination of services: a retirement system and better pay. The bill that established the U.S. Coast Guard also provided for the retirement of Sumner Increase Kimball, the man most responsible for the United States' excellent reputation for maritime rescue from shore-based stations.[6]

An immediate problem facing the new service in 1915 was how to integrate the Revenue Cutter Service and Life-Saving Service. This remained unsolved until the early 1960s, when all the organizations were finally combined into one. Until the United States entered World War II, for example, there were two types of districts within the service: a U.S. Coast Guard District, meaning cutters, and a Life-Saving District, meaning stations. One of the largest problems the merger caused, one that continues today, is the disconnect between the U.S. Revenue Cutter Service officer corps and the crews of the stations. In brief, when the two organizations merged, the U.S. Revenue Cutter Service had a corps of commissioned officers who received their education at a service academy. The people at the stations, on the other hand, were uneducated watermen who brought years of experience to their profession. As these watermen generally did not write anything but official reports, officers mistakenly felt there were no stories about the stations.

Eventually there developed an attitude among the leadership of the service that the stations could take care of themselves, with very little support, while the real work of the new service was in the cutter force. This attitude ceased only when the inevitable deaths at the stations occurred, or if there was a noteworthy rescue near budget time. If there was a death, officers investigated the cause, assigned blame, and made some suggestions, then business at the station continued as usual. All of this led those at the stations to expect very little in the way of newer equipment and people. The size of crews at the units, for example, changed very little from 1915 through the 1950s, although the caseloads steadily rose. The sense of being forgotten is still prevalent among those who serve at the stations. The leadership of the service has yet to fix this fault. Despite this, the crews who serve at the small boat rescue stations continue to push out into high seas to rescue those in distress.[7]

NEW BOATS

Twentieth-century technology brought many changes in maritime rescue from shore-based stations. By 1909, the U.S. Life-Saving Service had begun experimenting with gasoline engines in lifeboats. Not long after that, the service fitted surfboats with engines. No longer would human muscle have to battle the power of the sea. Lifeboatmen have always been a conservative lot, however. And with good reason. When you are battling fifteen- to twenty-foot breaking seas, that is not the time to have an as-yet-perfected piece of equipment fail. A veteran lifeboatman recalled old lifesavers telling him they would rather come across the bar with sail and oars than depend on a gasoline engine.

Despite reservations by the older lifeboatmen, in 1918 the U.S. Coast Guard introduced the 36-foot wooden motor lifeboat. The 36-footer, with some modifications, became the standard heavy weather boat of the service. From 1918 to 1937, the motor lifeboats still carried auxiliary sails, an indication of how the conservatism of the lifeboatmen still influenced the design of boats. Boats built after 1937 no longer carried sails. The U.S. Coast Guard Yard in Curtis Bay, Maryland, built a total of 281 lifeboats.[8]

The motor lifeboat was at best capable of nine miles per hour at full speed with a following sea. Lifeboatmen saw yachts literally running circles around their boat as it plodded steadily along. Yet when the weather worsened, the fancy yachts took to shelter or, more likely, called for help from the plodding but dependable 36-foot motor lifeboat. Looking at the motor lifeboats of the U.S. Coast Guard until 1964, one can see the basic lines of the English lifeboat of the 1870s. Despite the many modifications over the decades, the boats still offered little protection for the crew. In the words of an old salt, "You stood there and took the weather as it came at you." The only shelter was a canvas spray shield that often was difficult to raise, so there was no place to keep warm or dry. Many who worked on the boats felt that the boats would roll if so much as a turtle swam by. Most important, the 36-footer did exactly what it was designed to do: take generations of U.S. Coast Guardsmen out into gale-swept seas and bring them back safely.

The largest motor lifeboat in use from 1915 to 1964 was the 52-foot wooden craft introduced in 1935. Four steel-hulled lifeboats completed between 1956 and 1963 replaced the wooden craft. All four metal 52-footers are in service in the Pacific Northwest.[9] The U.S. Coast Guard also had other small craft of varying lengths. For sheltered waters, faster 30-foot and 40-foot utility boats augmented the motor lifeboats.[10]

FIXED-WING AVIATION

Following hard on the heels of the establishment of a new service, two visionary officers launched another method of providing maritime rescue. Lt. Elmer F. Stone and Lt. Norman B. Hall served on board the cutter *Onondaga* at Norfolk, Virginia. The two officers, in early 1915, requested that their commanding officer, Capt. Benjamin M. Chiswell, allow them to fly search missions for the cutter. Captain Chiswell approved the request. Stone and Hall next approached the Curtiss Flying School at Newport News, Virginia, with their idea. The officers flew experimental flights in the school's aircraft, using a Curtiss F flying boat as the platform for the experiment. The aircraft lacked navigational equipment, so it could not venture beyond the sight of land. Nevertheless, by the summer of 1916 the experiment had proved successful. Captain Commandant Ellsworth P. Bertholf sent Stone and five other officers to the U.S. Navy's aviation school at Pensacola, Florida. Hall received orders to the Curtiss factory to study aeronautical engineering. Later that same year, Congress authorized the U.S. Coast Guard to establish ten air stations along the seacoasts and Great Lakes. Money did not accompany the authority, and the plans for the stations died.[11]

During World War I, several U.S. Coast Guard aviators received orders to naval air stations at home and abroad, some in command positions. For example, Lt. Charles E. Sugden commanded the Île-Tudy Naval Air Station in France.[12] After the end of World War I, in March 1920, the U.S. Coast Guard established its first air station at Morehead City, North Carolina, at an abandoned naval air station. The service flew a few borrowed aircraft. Aircraft from Morehead City located those in distress and derelict ships that threatened navigation. This air station also fell for lack of funding on 1 July 1921.[13]

Prohibition, beginning in 1920, provided the impetus needed for the permanent establishment of U.S. Coast Guard aviation. In 1925, Lt. Cdr. Carl G. Von Paulsen borrowed a seaplane from the Navy and, operating out of Squantum, Massachusetts, and later Ten Pound Island in Gloucester Harbor, Massachusetts, demonstrated that aircraft were a powerful weapon against smugglers from the sea. Because of Von Paulsen's work, Congress finally funded the establishment of five air stations for the service.[14]

Although law enforcement was the determining factor in obtaining an aviation arm for the U.S. Coast Guard, the use of aircraft for search and rescue cases far offshore seemed obvious. In 1928, the service established an aviation section in headquarters, headed by Comdr. Norman B. Hall. To help mariners far offshore, the service developed the idea of the "flying lifeboat." These amphibian aircraft could fly many miles offshore and land in the open sea, but only in certain sea conditions.[15] In 1933, the ubiquitous Lieutenant Commander Von Paulsen showed both the strengths and weakness of seaplanes, becoming, in the process, one of the few commissioned U.S. Coast Guard aviation officers to win the coveted Gold Life Saving Medal.

THE ARCTURUS RESCUE

At about 11:30 A.M. on 1 January 1933, Station Chester Shoals, Florida, notified Air Station Miami of a missing boy. Paul Long had been blown offshore in a skiff just inside Cape Canaveral at 10:00 P.M. the previous night. The seaplane *Arcturus* was airborne at 12:20 P.M. with Lieutenant Commander Von Paulsen as pilot and Lt. William L. Foley as copilot. Other crew members were Chief Aviation Machinist Mate James R. Orndorff Jr., Aviation Machinist Mate 1st Class William D. Pinkston, and Radioman 3d Class Thomas S. McKenzie.[16]

Lieutenant Commander Von Paulsen flew through rainy, squally weather en route to the search area. Thirty miles southeast of Cape Canaveral, the aircrew located the skiff. Long "rose to his knees . . . and waved frantically" when he saw the aircraft. By this time Long was more than worried. Sharks followed the skiff. Each time a shark came too close, he struck at it with an oar. Von Paulsen put his seaplane in a wide circle, looking for craft that he could vector toward the skiff, but saw none.[17]

The nearest U.S. Coast Guard surface unit was eighty-five miles away. In an hour and a half the sun would set. As the aircraft passed over the skiff, the flight crew saw that Long and his boat were in poor shape. Adding to the situation, the squalls showed signs of increasing. Long carried no night signaling devices, which made it imperative to rescue him before nightfall.

In his official report, Von Paulsen related that he knew the only way to rescue Long was with an open sea landing.[18] The air crew lightened the seaplane by dumping surplus fuel. Dumping operations went wrong, however, and the gasoline sprayed back over the aircraft, seeping "through crevices and openings into the body" of the aircraft. The crew sprayed pyrene throughout the aircraft to prevent a fire. The mixture of the pyrene and gasoline caused the aircrew aft to become sick. Nevertheless, the enlisted flight crew worked on as they coughed and vomited. Von Paulsen later remarked that the fumes were not too bad "up front where I was, but the boys back aft certainly had a bad time of it."[19]

Von Paulsen lined up the aircraft for an open sea landing. Waves now reached twelve feet high, twice the height allowed for landing the aircraft in the open sea. When the plane set down, the impact caused the struts holding the left wing float to give way and the float banged against the wing. Von Paulsen ordered the flight crew out onto the right wing in an attempt to maintain an even keel.

McKenzie volunteered to enter the "darkening, rough, and shark-infested" water. When interviewed later, the radioman related, "I was in the water about ten or twelve minutes, the work of cutting away the wires went very slowly as I had only a pair of side-cutting pliers with which to cut the wires." The wires were too thick for the pliers. "The water was cold . . . and the seas rising and falling tossed me up and down. I had to hang on with one hand to prevent being swept away and I tore away at the wires with my free hand[,] meanwhile dodging the pounding pontoon which banged up and down with every crashing wave." In a remarkable bit of understatement, McKenzie said, "It was no fun!" He failed to mention that in the official report, Von Paulsen said that when McKenzie entered the water, he dived "directly above a shark." After cutting the wires, the radioman also swam to the skiff and brought Paul Long to the aircraft. Quickly, the crew hauled McKenzie and Long on board the damaged aircraft. Von Paulsen wrapped his flight jacket around the shivering radioman.[20]

Lieutenant Commander Von Paulsen now attempted to get his aircraft airborne. Pounding seas finally tore the pontoon off. Somehow he managed to get into the air, but he could not keep the damaged wing level; he made a forced landing on the sea. The seaplane struck the water so hard that its hull was damaged. Von Paulsen attempted to taxi the aircraft to shore, but this proved unsuccessful. Next he cut off the power to the engines and ordered a sea anchor deployed to keep the aircraft from turning sideways to the waves. Unfortunately, the line to the anchor carried away and the craft started to drift again.

After jury-rigging an antenna, McKenzie managed to get out an SOS. Meanwhile, the seaplane continued to drift until 1:00 A.M., when it passed through three lines of surf and beached inside a shoal. This allowed the crew to wade ashore, where they were found when help arrived. For their successful rescue, and despite many obstacles, the entire flight crew of the seaplane *Arcturus* received the Gold Life Saving Medal.[21]

HELICOPTERS

Although amphibious aircraft could make open sea landings, there was a limit to what they could accomplish, as illustrated by Von Paulsen's rescue. It was not until World War II, and as a result of the determination of two U.S. Coast Guard officers, that the service pioneered a better method. As with most innovations in a military organization, the path to success was a twisted one and one in which visionaries forfeited their careers to accomplish their dreams.

In the early morning hours of 7 December 1941, U.S. Coast Guard pilot Lt. Frank A. Erickson, on duty with the U.S. Navy, ran to his general quarters station in the aircraft control tower on Ford Island, Hawaii.[22] Erickson had "a grand view of the battle."[23] Helplessly, he witnessed the deaths of thousands of oil-drenched sailors desperately trying to struggle out of the sea. Among his many emotions on this "day of infamy" was frustration that U.S. Coast Guard aviation could do little to rescue these sailors.

Erickson then recalled an article he had read in *Aero Magazine* describing a small helicopter developed by Dr. Igor Sikorsky. Erickson grasped the importance of this new aircraft, and after that, his "greatest fear was not the war itself; it was that its duration would keep him in the Pacific unable to pursue his dream to effect a way to rescue victims at sea, using the Sikorsky helicopter."[24] From December 1941 onward, Erickson's sole purpose was to show the value of the helicopter in maritime rescue work.

Earlier, in 1938, Lt. Cdr. William Kossler had represented the U.S. Coast Guard on an interagency board for the evaluation of experimental aircraft, including the helicopter. Kossler understood the value of the aircraft and began working in headquarters for its adaption. An aviation historian points out that Kossler worked within the U.S. Coast Guard bureaucracy for adoption of the aircraft. Erickson, meanwhile, was the man in the field testing and using his ingenuity to perfect the helicopter for rescue work. Both officers were willing to risk their careers for this idea, and both died virtually unknown and with broken careers.[25]

Erickson's conviction caused many to look upon him as pushy. Capt. John M. Waters Jr., seagoing officer, pilot, and author, called him "a zealot (in the best sense of the word)."[26] Erickson looked like a football linebacker, and his appearance added force to his enthusiasm. His friends called him "Swede." Waters would later write, "Swede was always the salesman, willing to explain the helicopter's merits to anyone who would listen. His visions of the helicopter's future seemed highly extravagant to many of the fixed-wing clan, and his predictions were often ridiculed behind his back."[27]

In 1943, the U.S. Coast Guard received the task of developing the helicopter for antisubmarine warfare (ASW). Pilot training, under Erickson, began at the U.S. Coast Guard Air Station, Brooklyn, New York. During World War II, all Allied helicopter pilots received their training at this station.[28]

Erickson and Kossler continued their work convincing the service to accept the new aircraft. Commander Erickson became the first pilot to land on the deck of the cutter *Cobb*. As the war progressed, the service began to reorient its helicopter research to search and rescue. It was Erickson's drive and mind that developed many things that would make the helicopter an important tool in the war against the sea. He developed air-sea rescue methods and designed the first rescue hoist used to bring a person into a hovering helicopter. To make rescues easier, Erickson also designed a rescue basket hoisted by helicopter. Furthermore, he established a helicopter mechanic training program.[29] It seems only fitting that, true to his vision on that fateful day at Pearl Harbor, Erickson became the first helicopter pilot to fly a lifesaving mission.

On 3 January 1944, the U.S. Navy destroyer USS *Turner* lay anchored off Sandy Hook, New Jersey. A blizzard swept the area. Beginning at six o'clock in the morning, two powerful explosions, felt as far as fifteen miles away, racked the destroyer. Shortly after the second explosion, the ship sank. Ambulances brought many survivors into the hospital at Sandy Hook. The hospital desperately needed large quantities of plasma, but the roads and airfields were blocked due to the blizzard.

Adm. Stanley V. Parker, in command of U.S. Coast Guard activities in the Third Naval District, called Erickson "to ask if it would be practicable for a helicopter to pick up blood plasma at the [B]attery [in New York City] and fly it to Sandy Hook."[30] Here, at last, was Erickson's chance to prove his dream. If he felt any qualms about flying in such stormy conditions, he did not let it show. He responded to Admiral Parker with a loud "Yes, sir!" Shortly after receiving the telephone call, Erickson, along with Lt. (j.g.) Walter Bolton, prepared for their flight. Bolton had three whole days of helicopter qualification under his belt. Helicopter number 46445 lifted off, the aircraft disappearing "almost instantly" within low scudding clouds.

Erickson fought visibility so low that when he later recalled the mission he said, "We practically had to 'feel' our way around the ships anchored in Gravesend Bay." Buffeted by strong winds, he made a steep approach to Battery Park, near the southern tip of Manhattan Island. After landing, another problem developed. The weight of the two pilots plus the plasma was too much for the aircraft. Bolton reluctantly gave up his seat so the two cases of plasma could be strapped to the landing floats of the helicopter. Now Erickson faced another obstacle: trees blocked any chance for a forward takeoff. The "only way to get up was to back out," he recalled.

Erickson, fighting the wind, brought the aircraft slowly upward in vertical flight. As the helicopter shook, he maneuvered it backward out over the water and then spun it around and headed toward Sandy Hook. A few minutes later the helicopter landed with the plasma.

Later Erickson pointed out that given the "weather conditions," no other aircraft was capable of successfully completing this rescue. In the laconic manner perfected over the years by helicopter pilots, he went on to say that the flight was "routine for the helicopter." The *New York Times* disagreed. An editor noted that it "was indeed routine for the strange rotary-winged machine which Igor Sikorsky has brought to practical flight, but it shows in striking fashion how the helicopter makes use of tiny landing areas in conditions of visibility which make other types of flying impossible. . . . Nothing can dim the future of a machine which can take in its stride weather conditions such as those which prevailed on Monday." The first humanitarian mission of the helicopter took all of fourteen minutes.

LABRADOR

The first major rescue by a U.S. Coast Guard helicopter took place in Canada. On 19 April 1945, a Royal Canadian Air Force twin-engine PBY-5A patrol aircraft on a flight from Iceland suffered severe icing. Initially, one engine quit; shortly after that, the other engine stopped. The aircraft broke out of the clouds above mountain peaks in Labrador, just north of Anticosti Island. The pilot managed to put the crippled PBY into clumps of spruce trees, which saved the nine crewmen. Unfortunately, the trees also ripped open the airplane upon landing. Crewmen quickly removed their survival gear from the wrecked patrol aircraft. As the men worked, leaking fuel ignited, burning two crewmen and destroying the aircraft.[31]

The crew began treating the burned men and building a survival camp. An inventory of their supplies revealed enough rations for eight days. Some men tramped out letters in the snow that read "SOS" and "MO" (medical officer) on a nearby frozen pond. Others built signal smoke fires with green tree limbs. While the survivors huddled in their cold camp, a massive search was set in motion. No sooner had the search begun, than a two-day blizzard halted all operations. Once the weather lifted, twenty-two aircraft resumed the search. All aircraft transiting the route of the missing aircraft also looked for any sign of the missing PBY.

Although the downed crew saw some searching aircraft, those conducting the search did not see the survivor's camp. Three days of disappointment drove the PBY's crew to a desperate decision. An overland party, with five days of rations, would strike out in the hope of crossing the ninety miles to Goose Bay. On the first day of the trek, everything changed for the better. A cargo aircraft spotted both the camp and those trying to make their way overland.

Soon after that, two single-engine ski-equipped aircraft appeared over the survivors. One landed on the trail of the overland party, took the men on board, and then lifted off. It crashed, but there were no injuries. The other aircraft landed near the camp and took off with the burned men.

Nine men remained in the cold survival camp. The single-engine aircraft brought in additional supplies for the survivors. Bad weather again swept the area, and two days passed before single-engine ski planes could reach the crash location. Some survivors were loaded into the aircraft. When the skiplanes tried to take off, however, their skis stuck in the mushy snow. The crews threw out everything possible and managed to lift off with only four survivors on board. Spring thaw was on, and no other ski plane, or dogsled, could get into the site. There were only two alternatives: wait until everything melted and try to get a floatplane to land on a nearby lake (this would require many weeks) or wait until the next winter for ski planes.

This was a situation made for Erickson's helicopter. There was only one helicopter "marginally" capable of performing the rescue mission, but it was not available as it was conducting experiments in ASW work. There was also a trainer available at Floyd Bennett Field in Brooklyn. This aircraft had a very short range and able to take only one survivor on board at a time. The solution to the problem illustrates that the small boat community of the U.S. Coast Guard does not hold a license on ingenuity.

Mechanics disassembled the rescue helicopter, an HNS from Floyd Bennet Field, and loaded it into a C-54 cargo plane of the Air Transport Command at Floyd Bennett. The C-54 lifted off with helicopter and U.S. Coast Guard crew on board. The aircraft arrived at Goose Bay on 29 April. Crews immediately set about reassembling the helicopter and finished their work the next morning.

Lt. August Kleisch, U.S. Coast Guard, lifted off with the float-equipped aircraft. He carried seven five-gallon jerry cans of gasoline strapped to the floats for the 184-mile flight to Lake Mecatina via the survivors camp. The distance was 30 percent farther than the normal range of the helicopter. A PBY circled above the helicopter to escort the slower moving aircraft.

About halfway to the survivors, Kleisch landed on a lake to refuel the helicopter from the gas cans. Ten feet of snow lay on the lake. While the aircraft did not break through the crust of the snow, Lieutenant Kleisch did, sinking up to his hips. Kleisch later related that the area "was a desolate and eerie sight, the heavy silence broken only by the comforting sound of the PBY as it circled overhead. Getting back in the air was a relief."

Soon after that, the helicopter landed at the survivors' camp. The downed airmen "cheered" as the strange aircraft landed. After accepting a cup of coffee and again refueling the aircraft, Lieutenant Kleisch took on board his first passenger, Sgt. G. J. Bunnell. When he tried to lift off, the pilot found the floats frozen in the snow. Kleisch had to make a "jump takeoff" by overspeeding the engines and "giving the blades all the pitch" he could. The U.S. Coast Guard officer noted that Sergeant Bunnell at first was nervous about flying in this new aircraft and "continually looked up apprehensively at the rotor blades." Bunnell settled down after the helicopter cleared the tree tops.

With Kleisch and Bunnell on board, the helicopter barely made fifty miles per hour. Kleisch's destination was an isolated radio range station at Mecantina Lake, about thirty-eight miles east of the crash site. The nine Canadian Air Force enlisted men stationed at this extremely isolated location rejoiced so much at seeing other people that Kleisch later said it was difficult to know who was happier, the downed aircrew or the radio station crew. To speed up the rescue, a PBY earlier had dropped barrels of gasoline from the air to refuel the helicopter, but the entire load had broken upon impact. There was, however, some gasoline stored under the ice at the station. The station's crew dug out the supply and helped strain it through chamois cloths and used it to refuel the helicopter and fill jerry cans.

During the first night at the station, the thermometer dropped to ten degrees Fahrenheit, freezing the helicopter's engine. A single-engine aircraft the next morning brought in a heater, and a U.S. Coast Guard aviation machinist mate, to thaw the engine. Soon, the helicopter began bringing out one survivor at a time. The single-engine aircraft then shuttled the men to Goose Bay. Finally, on 2 May, after nine trips, the last of the downed airmen reached safety.

"SWEDE" VERSUS THE MAN WITH A CIGAR

Today the public sees the helicopter as the U.S. Coast Guard's mainstay in aviation maritime rescues. It may be difficult to grasp that until the 1960s within the service there was great resistance to rotary-wing aircraft. The leadership of the U.S. Coast Guard felt that amphibious fixed-wing aircraft was best for the service. There developed within the service a strong rift between the two groups. Commissioned officers who chose the wrong side found their careers finished, and the wrong side was in helicopters.

A leading proponent of fixed-wing aircraft was one of those colorful people who seem to populate any history of maritime search and rescue. Donald Bartram MacDiarmid was the second son of a Methodist minister who graduated in 1929 from the U.S. Coast Guard Academy "through the Grace of God and somebody's mistake." Before attending the academy, he had served a short period as an enlisted man in the U.S. Navy. Some viewed him as a "true hero" who "epitomized in real life the type often portrayed by the movie idol John Wayne." Few retired enlisted men, however, have spoken with fondness about their experience of serving under the officer.[32]

MacDiarmid, after completing a year of sea duty, went through Navy flight training and, almost unbelievably, failed his final flight and "washed out." Later speculation would have it that the failure was due more to his belligerence toward instructors than his flying abilities. After washing out, he received orders to a 125-foot cutter. "Sea stories" relate that after MacDiarmid's first patrol, the entire deck force deserted the cutter, except one man. When investigators asked this lone seaman why he remained, his reply was that he had "only five days left in the Coast Guard."[33]

No one now seems to know why, but somehow MacDiarmid received a second chance at flight school and graduated in April 1938. Interestingly, his first duty at an air station was as commanding officer, the only position he held at various air stations throughout the rest of his long career.[34]

Even many of MacDiarmid's detractors do not deny his focused intensity when it came to saving lives at sea. He expected his crews to either run or use a bicycle to quickly reach the ready aircraft when the SAR alarm rang. If a pilot was a little late, he would find MacDiarmid sitting in the pilot's seat. At the Port Angeles, Washington, air station, MacDiarmid kept a bicycle by the door of the administration building. When the SAR alarm blasted, he ran down the stairs, leaped astride the bicycle, and peddled to the ready aircraft. He once flew into a rage when someone stole his bicycle. (A bicycle still stands ready, bearing a stenciled sign "CO's," near the door of the Port Angeles air station's administration building.) Another time the SAR alarm rang and the ready crew beat MacDiarmid to the aircraft and, once inside, locked the doors. As the amphibious craft rolled down the launching ramp, the ground crew observed their commanding officer running alongside, pounding on its side and only giving up his efforts when the plane entered the water.[35]

MacDiarmid placed people into two categories; they were "eager rescue pilots or they weren't. If you were in the former, you could do little wrong. If not, things were rocky. Flying came first and paperwork second. Nothing interfered with SAR."[36]

Capt. John M. Waters Jr. recalled when MacDiarmid received orders to Washington, D.C., to sit on a personnel board headed by a rear admiral. "Mac considered [the admiral] to be a 'first rate clerk.'" MacDiarmid walked into the board room for the first meeting carrying a brown paper bag. The admiral, aloofly, said, "Captain, why are you bringing your lunch? In the big city, we have restaurants."

" 'I don't have lunch in the bag,' replied MacDiarmid, placing it carefully on the green covered table.

" 'Oh?' said the great man, obviously curious.

" 'No sir. Before this board is over, I'll probably want to puke. The bag is for that.' "[37]

One historian noted that MacDiarmid studied the sea and worked on methods that would lead to safer means for aircraft ditching at sea. Beginning in 1943, and continuing for the next three years, MacDiarmid conducted seaplane test operations in the open sea near San Diego, California. Many results of his studies and experiments are still in use. For his work, MacDiarmid received the Distinguished Flying Cross from the U.S. Navy. One contemporary wrote that although MacDiarmid was "single minded, controversial, and with a zealot's drive, [he] was the man who more than any other made the seaplane and rough water compatible."[38]

At the end of World War II, the U.S. Coast Guard had two very strong personalities and dreamers as advocates for the type of aircraft that would be used in rescue at sea. Erickson saw the helicopter as the answer. MacDiarmid felt the seaplane was the best method.

In the 1950s, as more SAR cases involved recreational boaters, the value of the helicopter became more evident. The 1950s also brought much publicity to the helicopters of the U.S. Coast Guard in flood work. In 1955, for example, the service's helicopters rescued more than 300 people as rivers overflowed their banks in Connecticut and Massachusetts. In December of that year, one HO4S U.S. Coast Guard helicopter rescued 138 people in a twelve-hour period at Yuba City, California, by using two air crews.[39]

MacDiarmid, "always a realist," realized that helicopters were taking over much of the SAR work.[40] In a June 1953 letter, he wrote, "So many boys have been busting these mechanized Pogo sticks—and a few killing themselves in the operation—I decided inasmuch as I have to order people out in these things I'd better learn to fly them myself."[41] He qualified in helicopters on 11 June 1953 and, predictably, quickly became the target of those on whom he had at one time heaped scorn. One of his fellow officers wrote a note that sums up what many felt: "I hear via the grapevine that you are now a helicrapper [*sic*] pilot, and have conceded that Erickson was right all along. We have heard rumors that the ready spot at the ramp is now occupied by a HO4S instead of a PBM [seaplane]."[42]

MacDiarmid continued, even as a commanding officer and at the age of forty-seven, to stand SAR duty and still raced junior officers to the ready aircraft. One historian notes that it really "was not the type of plane that mattered to the man."[43]

The early 1960s marked the beginning of the end of seaplanes in the U.S. Coast Guard. The aircraft's excessive weight, operational inflexibility, and inability to continuously perform open sea landings helped in its demise.[44] In the end, Erickson proved correct.

Erickson reached the rank of captain and retired early. Except for one brief tour, the leadership of the service never allowed him to hold a command. Disillusioned, he felt he had failed to promote the helicopter and had received no recognition for his contributions. Although discouraged, he never gave up his dream. In 1969, he wrote his brother that "Coast Guard aviation will be an all helicopter outfit before long except for a few land planes used for logistic purposes."[45] Capt. Frank Erickson died in December 1978 and lived to see his prophecy come true.

MacDiarmid retired in 1959. Unlike Erickson, MacDiarmid held a number of aviation commands. Again unlike Erickson, MacDiarmid received some measure of fame when he received the Distinguished Flying Cross. Capt. Donald B. MacDiarmid died in November 1980.

7 | Business as Usual

New weapons and a new name brought very little change in the constant war against the sea fought by the crews of the U.S. Coast Guard's rescue stations. The daily routines and crew sizes at U.S. Coast Guard lifeboat stations up to 1964 were much the same as those of the U.S. Life-Saving Service. Although twentieth-century technology allowed ships to remain farther off shore, the stations continued drilling with the beach apparatus. Especially during the early years of the twentieth century, crews still put the equipment to use.

Within the first twenty-nine years of the U.S. Coast Guard's existence, two world wars dominated international events. At first glance it would seem that the United States' entry into World Wars I and II would change everything for the small boat rescue stations. Crews, however, still faced the struggle with the sea. A global war dominated newspaper headlines in 1918, but two events illustrate how small boat rescue stations continued their traditional duty.

ABOVE THE FALLS

At 3:30 P.M. on 6 August 1918, the watchstander at the U.S. Coast Guard lifeboat station at Fort Niagara (Niagara Station), New

York, received a telephone call. The caller reported that "two men had been carried into the rapids just above the brink of [Niagara Falls] in a mud scow."[1] Warrant Officer Albert D. Nelson, the commanding officer of Niagara Station, knew that dredging operations were underway on the Niagara River along the New York–Canadian border. Nelson learned the tug *Hassayampa*, towing a mud barge, had run aground. A second tug had managed to pull *Hassayampa* free, only to have the towline part. With no tow or power, the barge headed downstream for the Horseshoe Falls portion of Niagara Falls, with Gustaf Loftberg and James Harris on board. In a desperate move to ground the barge, the two men opened the seacocks to let in the water and threw out an anchor.

Somehow the barge entered a rocky area, instead of the main channel a few feet away, and ran aground. It rested about 150 yards above the falls and about a thousand feet from the Canadian shoreline. Attempts to reach the men with a shoulder-fired shotline rifle failed. Warrant Officer Nelson arranged for a "motor truck" from Fort Niagara to load the beach apparatus, "with a lot of extra lines," plus transport six soldiers and two surfmen. Nelson and two surfmen followed in Nelson's automobile.

Maritime lifesavers of both the U.S. Life-Saving Service and U.S. Coast Guard have overcome many obstacles while saving lives. On this case, Nelson would face some highly unusual problems not usually experienced in the annals of the service. The small convoy started south on a fourteen-mile journey to the site of the barge. After making an unexpected detour, the convoy finally approached and stopped at the bridge to the Canadian border. A "flap . . . arose about rushing a cannon across the bridge under wartime security."[2] Nelson managed to convince officials he was on a humanitarian mission and not intent on invading Canada. The delays caused the lifesavers to reach the scene at 4:25 P.M., fifty-five minutes after receiving the telephone call.

Nelson estimated the barge lay fourteen hundred feet from the shore. In his report on the incident, he wrote, "We immediately shot a line over [to] the scow." Loftberg and Harris began pulling the smaller lines over to the barge. Nelson, along with surfmen, soldiers, and other volunteers, managed to work the lines and equipment to the "roof of the General Electric building, 10 or 12 stories high, in order to keep the lines out of the swift current."

The barge had no mast, so Loftberg and Harris had to laboriously pull everything over by hand instead of using a block and tackle. This proved too much for them and they set about rigging up a windlass. "It took them nearly two hours" to get the device to pull over the heavy rope hawser, "which also was slow work on account of the current." Once the hawser finally reached the barge and Loftberg and Harris made it fast, they had to haul away the breeches buoy. The sun had now set and darkness added to the difficulties. The lines continually fouled, adding to the exhaustion of both men, who also suffered from the drenching spray thrown by the falls. The noise from the falls likewise prevented communication during the rescue, making the already complicated situation worse.

One account reports that William "Red" Hill, "a Niagara resident" who was "home from France recovering from the effects of war wounds and poison gas," volunteered to attempt to free the lines. Hill "crawled out onto the snarled lines and himself became entangled, dangling inches above the rapids. Working himself free, he got the lines operational."[3]

Nelson sent over the breeches buoy with written instructions. The two sailors rigged everything and awaited daylight. Dawn brought light to the scene. Loftberg and Harris came ashore within forty-five minutes of rigging the breeches buoy. A doctor treated both for exhaustion and then released them.

Lines from the beach apparatus work "trailed out over the falls for months." As of 2004, the barge remains where it grounded above Horseshoe Falls.[4] The lifesavers did not return to their station until 1:30 P.M. the next day, having spent more than twenty-one hours saving two men from certain death.

THE BLAZING SEA

Four days after Warrant Officer Albert D. Nelson's struggle at Niagara Falls, there occurred a rescue that included one of the worse fears of sailors: fire. In the second week of August 1918, Warrant Officer John Allen Midgett commanded the Chicamacomico Station on the Outer Banks of North Carolina. Midgett knew better than most Americans that World War I now encompassed the eastern shore of the United States. During the prior week, on Tuesday, 5 August, for example, a German U-boat had sunk a Dutch ship, the *Diamond Shoals* lightship, and had forced two steamers aground with fire from its deck gun.[5] Midgett, on 11 August 1918, would come face to face with both the war with the sea and the Germans.

John Allen Midgett brought experience and family tradition to what would become known in the annals of the U.S. Coast Guard as the *Mirlo* case. The Midgett family of the Outer Banks has served in the U.S. Coast Guard and its predecessors since at least 1874. One Midgett observed that on the Outer Banks "you could either sit around and fish, or you could go out and save lives" and the family chose the latter.[6] On 11 August, John Allen Midgett possessed eighteen years of experience at the stations along the Outer Banks. Locals called him "Captain Johnny," and his crew addressed him as "Captain." Midgett would need all the experience, family tradition, and guts he could muster before the day was over.[7]

The making of a legend within the U.S. Coast Guard began when Capt. William Roose Williams ordered the British tanker *Mirlo* underway from New Orleans, Louisiana, on Saturday, 10 August 1918. The 6,997-ton tanker shipped fifty-two sailors and carried a cargo of gasoline and oil. *Mirlo* rounded Cape Hatteras, North Carolina, on Friday, the sixteenth. Shortly after noon the tanker approached the Wimble Shoals Light Buoy.[8]

As *Mirlo* approached the buoy, the German submarine *U-117* lay submerged about thirteen hundred feet away. Kapitanleutnant Droscher watched through the U-boat's periscope as the ship approached. At 3:30 P.M., at a range of 1,308 feet, Droscher gave the order to fire a torpedo, set to run at a depth of three meters (nine feet, ten inches), from tube number 1. Through the periscope, Droscher viewed a large explosion.[9]

On board *Mirlo,* the explosion engulfed the engine room, causing the loss of lights and radio communications. Captain Williams ordered his crew to run out the lifeboats while he attempted to beach his ship. Shortly after that, a second explosion racked the ship. Williams gave the order to abandon ship. Second Mate J. Burns, with fourteen of the crew on board, got the first lifeboat away, but it capsized. The crewmen managed to reach and cling to the overturned lifeboat. Two other lifeboats managed to get safely away. One, commanded by First Mate F. J. Campbell, started toward the sailors in the water. Suddenly a third explosion rocked the area, spewing burning cargo out onto the water. The sea was now a blazing inferno of gasoline and oil.[10]

The towering fire separated Captain Williams's boat from the others. "We were almost burning and it was only by the strenuous efforts on the oars that we managed to save our lives, the fire following us within a few feet for half an hour at least," Williams later recalled. He was sure the rest of his crew had perished.[11]

Once clear of the fire, Williams called for his sailors, despite suffering from shock and burns, "to lay on their oars." In the tradition of the sea, Williams felt he must at least try to see if any of his crew survived. At just this moment, the captain sighted a boat on the horizon making toward his lifeboat. It was the powered, self-bailing surfboat from Chicamacomico Station.[12]

Earlier, Surfman Leroy Midgett, standing the lookout tower watch at Chicamacomico Station, spotted a ship to the southeast. While he watched, he saw an explosion slightly aft of amidship and a large geyser of water shoot upward. Surfman Midgett gave the alarm. Captain Johnny immediately recalled all hands. The crew ran to the stables and hitched horses to the boat wagon on which rested a 20-foot, 4-inch Beebe-McLellan motor self-bailing surfboat, number 1046.

The lifesavers quickly transported the boat six hundred yards from the station to the water's edge and launched into breakers eighteen to twenty feet high. Three times the boat swamped. Finally, on the fourth try, the small craft cleared the surf zone and entered the rough open sea. Midgett noted the time: 5:00 P.M.[13]

John Allen Midgett's boat carried many of the Midgett family that day. LeRoy Midgett was one of the smaller members of the station, with light blue eyes and an oval face. Zion S. Midgett, powerfully built, joined the service before the turn of the twentieth century. Arthur V. Midgett was prematurely gray, with a ruddy complexion, of medium height, with broad shoulders and a thick chest. Clarence E. Midgett, at more than six feet tall, towered above the entire crew. He was slender, with brown hair, blue eyes, and a medium complexion. The only crewmember who was not a member of the Midgett family was thirty-eight-year-old Prochorus L. O'Neal, known as Lee, who was five feet ten inches tall. These six Outer Banks lifesavers would shortly set into motion a rescue that has become an icon in the tradition of maritime lifesaving in the United States.[14]

When Captain Johnny's surfboat reached *Mirlo*'s lifeboat, the keeper raised a speaking trumpet and hailed Captain Williams. Midgett asked if they needed assistance. Williams requested Midgett "to go to the rescue of one boat capsized and one boat intact with part of my crew in it." The two boats were now five miles offshore. Before starting toward *Mirlo*, Captain Johnny warned Williams to remain outside the surf zone unless other help arrived. Williams and his British seaman watched as the six lifesavers and their power surfboat headed toward the blazing sea. Within minutes, the U.S. Coast Guard boat and crew disappeared from view in the smoke.[15]

Within several hundred yards of *Mirlo*, Midgett found the tanker in two parts, with about seventy-five feet of water between the bow and the stern. The bow being the closest, John Allen Midgett maneuvered toward it. As he closed on the bow, barrels of gasoline continued to explode on board *Mirlo*. As each barrel detonated, flames shot hundreds of feet into the air. The surface of the sea between the surfboat and the bow was an inferno. As the surfboat neared the flames, LeRoy Midgett yelled to Captain Johnny that he thought he saw the periscope of a U-boat.[16]

Undaunted, John Allen Midgett circled the blazing hulk, looking for an opening in the blazing sea. On the lee side, Midgett found an opening. The smoke cleared enough for the boat crew to see two giant pillars of fire. Near the bow of *Mirlo,* Midgett spied the tanker's overturned lifeboat, buffeted by heavy swells. At first, Midgett saw no survivors around the overturned craft, but he steered "through the smoke, floating wreckage, and burning gas and oil" toward the lifeboat. As his surfboat chugged along, the U.S. Coast Guardsmen saw a flaming arch and through the arch a man clinging to the lifeboat. Approaching closer, the lifesaving crew now saw other survivors clinging to the lifeboat's gunwales. Only six of the fifteen remained alive, having survived by constantly ducking beneath the sea.[17]

Midgett and his crew pulled the burned, oil-coated sailors from the sea. The heat from the fire scorched and blistered the paint on the motor surfboat. In a classic understatement, LeRoy Midgett later said it was "hot country." Nevertheless, the U.S. Coast Guardsmen searched the immediate area for other survivors. This proved futile. The lifesavers now began searching for the missing lifeboat of First Mate Campbell.[18]

John Allen Midgett concluded that the missing lifeboat might be downwind from the tanker and headed in that direction. Nine miles southeast of Chicamacomico, the lifesavers found the boat. Midgett took the craft in tow and made for the location where Captain Williams should be waiting outside the surf zone.[19]

Darkness was setting in when Captain Williams saw the U.S. Coast Guard motor surfboat towing one of his ship's lifeboats. At first, the survivors in William's lifeboat thought that everyone in *Mirlo*'s crew was safe and the British sailors give "a loud cheer." Joy quickly turned to sadness, however, when Midgett announced "a number of lives had been lost."[20]

Captain Johnny took Captain Williams's boat in tow and started toward Hatteras Island. Within two miles of Chicamacomico, the wind freshened. Midgett ordered *Mirlo*'s lifeboats anchored outside the surf zone. He then took his motor surfboat, with the six survivors pulled from water, through the surf into the shore. Citizens from the surrounding area and the U.S. Coast Guard crew from Gull Shoal to the north illuminated the shore with lights. They helped in taking the burned and oily sailors to shelter. John Allen Midgett and his crew again headed out into the surf.[21]

Midgett steered to *Mirlo*'s lifeboats. The lifesavers transferred some survivors to the motor surfboat. Captain Johnny and his crew shuttled four loads of survivors to the beach. On the last trip out, U.S. Coast Guardsmen went on board the now empty *Mirlo* lifeboats and then beached the craft. The last survivor came ashore at 9:00 P.M. After securing the boats on the beach, John Allen Midgett returned to Chicamacomico Station and closed his log at 11:00.[22]

In a letter to his company, Captain Williams wrote that "the eyes of all the life saving crew were all bloodshot, which was caused by their getting so close to the fire as to be partly gassed and smoke into their eyes." Further, the lifesavers had "done one of the bravest deeds which I have seen."[23] John Allen Midgett and his entire boat crew received the Gold Life Saving Medal and a special medal from King George V, and the British Board of Trade gave John Midgett a silver cup. Nine years after the rescue, on 23 July 1930, John Allen Midgett and his crew received Grand Crosses of the American Cross of Honor, presented to them by the commandant of the U.S. Coast Guard, Rear Adm. Frederick C. Billard.[24]

John Allen Midgett went on to serve in the U.S. Coast Guard for another twenty years, retiring with a total of thirty-eight years of service. "He participated in 40 major rescues and in hundreds of smaller ones."[25] The man who escaped the flames of the torpedoed *Mirlo* and other dangerous rescues at sea would die in an automobile accident two days before Christmas 1937. He lies in the family plot at Manteo, North Carolina.[26]

RESCUE OF THE *H. E. RUNNELS*

During the closing days of the 1919 shipping season on Lake Superior, the 178-foot, 889-ton steamer *H. E. Runnels* left Buffalo, New York, bound for Lake Linden, in upper Michigan's

Keeweenaw Peninsula, with a cargo of coal. When off Grand Marais, Michigan, about one hundred miles east of its destination, the steamer ran into one of Lake Superior's infamous northwesters. Capt. Hugh O'Hagan wisely sought the shelter of Grand Marais's harbor.[27]

The next morning, 14 November 1919, Captain O'Hagan felt the storm had abated enough to continue his voyage. Shortly afterward, *Runnels* entered Lake Superior. O'Hagan soon realized the northwester had not yet released Lake Superior from its grip. Staring through the bridge's ports at snow driven by sixty knots of howling wind, he ordered *Runnels* back to the safe shelter of Grand Marais.[28]

Driving snow made the visibility poor. O'Hagan ordered his ship at the slowest maneuverable speed possible. Even with very little way on, *Runnels* missed the harbor entrance. O'Hagan ordered the helm hard over, trying to work the steamer back into Lake Superior and another approach to the harbor. The rudder controls failed. *Runnels,* now rudderless, faced a fate dependent upon the driving winds and seas; it struck 150 feet from the outer end of the west pier.[29]

Meanwhile, *Runnels*'s plight had not gone unnoticed at the U.S. Coast Guard lifeboat station at Grand Marias. The station's lookout, George Olsen, about a quarter of a mile southeast of the wreck, at 5:30 A.M. reported a steamer on the "wrong side of the west pier at the harbor entrance."[30] Thinking that the steamer was standing into danger, Olsen prudently rang the station's alarm. The crew quickly prepared the beach apparatus and then launched their boat.

From the tower, Olsen noticed the ship back out into the lake and hove to. The still-unknown ship showed no distress signals. Normally, Benjamin Trudell, the commanding officer, would have been the man making decisions at the Grand Marais Station. A longtime keeper on Lake Superior and first keeper of the station when it opened in 1900, Trudell knew his business. Frederick T. Stonehouse, a historian of shipwrecks on Lake Superior, notes that Trudell was "a living legend along the south shore of Lake

Superior" and that his knowledge and leadership "was an important ingredient in the station's success."[31] On 14 November, however, Trudell was ill and Surfman Number 1 Alfred E. Kristofferson was in charge.

Kristofferson felt the steamer would lie off the harbor and await daylight before making another attempt to enter it. Like many old lifesavers who knew their profession, Kristofferson prepared for the worse. The first problem he faced was the fact that many of his surfmen were sick and he needed extra men if he had to launch the boat.

As fate would have it, a U.S. Coast Guard cutter, the 110-foot former sub chaser *SC-438*, happened to be sheltering in the harbor. The cutter, en route to Minnesota, sought refuge from the storm.[32] Kristofferson walked over to the *438* to speak to the commanding officer, Lt. G. R. O'Connor, about obtaining help from his crew. O'Connor agreed to help as much as possible. Again, in another of those fateful happenings, O'Connor mentioned he had a guest aboard the cutter, John O. Anderson, a veteran keeper from the station at Chicago, Illinois. Would Kristofferson accept Anderson's help, if needed? Kristofferson readily accepted the offer.[33]

When Kristofferson and Anderson reached the station, they learned the motor lifeboat was not running. After Olsen had heard the *Runnels*'s horn signaling distress, the station crew launched the motor lifeboat and started to the *SC-438* to pick up Kristofferson. The engine failed. Unable to restart it, the crew anchored and waded ashore. With the lifeboat out of commission, the next method Anderson and Kristofferson focused upon was the beach apparatus.[34]

The U.S. Coast Guardsmen arrived at the scene. They observed *Runnels* lying broadside to high, choppy seas. A combination of seas breaking over the pier and the steamer made a "nasty cross sea," with spray filling the air. The thermometer hovered at eighteen degrees below zero Fahrenheit. Spray quickly froze to any surface. Driving snow made it nearly impossible to make out the steamer. Incredibly, despite the fierce conditions, there stood the almost inevitable group of spectators. Scattered among the onlookers were the wives of the U.S. Coast Guardsmen who would push off into this terrible sea. Also among the bystanders were some men who would play a role in the rescue.[35]

Anderson quickly took over. He ordered the beach apparatus rigged then loaded, aimed, and fired the Lyle gun. The shotline flew over *Runnels*'s bowsprit. "It was . . . a shot that had to be made, since the bow was the only area not either under water or being regularly swept by the waves."[36] Sailors aboard the steamer hauled out the block. So far, Anderson and the other U.S. Coast Guardsmen had followed procedures as laid down by U.S. Coast Guard regulations for beach apparatus rescue. As all too often happens in maritime rescue cases, another problem arose. As the sailors aboard *Runnels* hauled in the block, the ice-coated lines fouled and could not be freed. This forced Anderson to come up with a third plan of attack.[37]

Kristofferson suggested that since the whipline was aboard *Runnels,* perhaps they could jury-rig something with the surfboat. The surfman thought that by doubling the line that ran from *Runnels* to the beach, it could guide the surfboat. Anderson agreed. Soon the crew rammed the surfboat into the heavy seas.[38]

Anderson, in the stern of the boat, used his sweep oar to keep the pitching, rolling craft within the confines of the jury-rigged lines. Eight men, made up of station crew, volunteers from *SC-438,* and one volunteer fisherman, pulled at the oars. Spray and waves lashed the lifesavers. The water froze on the faces and hands of the rescuers. Some crewmembers found themselves thrown from the boat into churning Lake Superior. In a display of "exceptional steering and oarmanship," the small boat came alongside *Runnels.*[39] The lifesavers tried to throw a line to the sailors on the ship. The actions of the small boat were so violent that the crew aboard *Runnels* could not catch the line. Now the lifesavers had to convince the sailors to work their way down the line from the beach apparatus hand over hand and into the boat.

One of the most dangerous times in a rescue is when a shipwrecked crew must enter a small boat. Ingrained into the memories of all those in the service is what could happen if a crew panics and leaps at the same time. In 1876, for example, the crew of the Italian ship *Nuova Ottavia* panicked and leaped at once, crashing into the lifesaver's boat and drowning both crews. Seven lifesavers were lost.[40]

Four of *Runnels*'s crew made their way down the line one at a time, into the pitching rolling boat. Anderson, knowing that the rowing and holding station near *Runnels* had taken its toll in his crew's strength, ordered his crew to pull back to the beach. Once safely landed, Anderson found his crew suffering from exhaustion and exposure. Two U.S. Coast Guardsmen were carried away with "cramps and suffering from exposure."[41] Two brothers, Ambose and Joseph Graham, volunteered to replace the two lifesavers. Both knew how to handle an oar, as they had served in the U.S. Life-Saving Service.[42] Anderson again ordered the boat into Lake Superior. Volunteers replaced the exhausted men each of the three times the boat returned to the beach. One man, Ora Endress, braved the lake three times.[43]

On the fourth, and final, trip in the small boat, only Captain O'Hagan and his first mate were aboard *Runnels*. By this time, there were no more volunteers available. Anderson set out into the tempest with an undermanned boat of six instead of the normal eight.[44]

Reaching *Runnels* after a difficult pull, Anderson and his lifesavers faced yet another problem: the first mate awaiting rescue weighed at least three hundred pounds. To say this spelled trouble is to understate on a grand scale. Anderson, in another example of lifesavers' on-the-spot improvisation, had Captain O'Hagan and his first mate tie lines around their waists before making the difficult transition to the small rescue boat.[45]

The extra lines proved their salvation. Both O'Hagan and the mate fell into the frigid, churning waters, but the lifesavers managed to get the lines and started to pull the two men into the boat. Another problem developed, however. The weight of the mate caused the boat to ship water and throw some rescuers into the lake. Somehow the fatigued crew managed to reach the safety of the beach. The last surfboat reached *Runnels* at 12:40 P.M. Thirty minutes later, the steamer broke up. All seventeen sailors aboard the steamer reached safety.[46]

The work at *Runnels* took a heavy toll on the U.S. Coast Guardsmen. The seas threw Anderson out of the boat at least four times. Kristofferson twice found himself in Lake Superior.[47] Capt. O'Connor, although the senior U.S. Coast Guard officer present, should have taken command of the rescue. O'Connor, however, knew who the experts were and let Anderson and Kristofferson take over the rescue. After the rescue, however, O'Connor ordered Kristofferson relieved of any responsibility for the equipment still on the beach and directly to the station for recovery.[48]

Due to the courage of the lifesavers and their ability to improvise under dire conditions, no one died on this stormy January morning in 1919. All who ventured out into the stormy lake received the Gold Life Saving Medal.[49]

RESCUE OF THE *TRINIDAD*

Hilman John Persson was born on 3 September 1888 in Sweden. At the age of eighteen, sponsored by his uncle Mattis Persson, Hillman immigrated to the United States in 1906. Mattis Persson was a surfman at the U.S. Life-Saving Service station at Gray's Harbor, Washington, about thirty miles north of the dangerous Columbia River. When Hilman arrived at Gray's Harbor, he could not speak English.[50]

Like many in the Pacific Northwest at the time, Hilman worked in the timber industry. Dissatisfied with that profession, he followed Mattis's advice and signed on as a temporary surfman at the Gray's Harbor Station. Hilman substituted whenever a surfman became sick, or had a family emergency. The keeper recognized Hilman's abilities in a boat and hired him as a full-time surfman in 1907.[51] "At the time I joined the lifesaving service," Persson would later recall, "none of the boats at the station were equipped with motors because no dependable small gasoline motor had been invented yet, and besides we were always slow in receiving up-to-date equipment. We, the oarsmen of the station,

considered ourselves fortunate because, in going to the assistance
of a vessel in distress, there was nearly always a seagoing steam tug
at the Westport dock that we could depend on towing us to the
scene . . . Unfortunately there were many times when there was no
tug available."[52]

Hilman remained in the U.S. Life-Saving Service and became
a part of the new U.S. Coast Guard in 1915. At the age of thirty,
in 1919, he transferred to the station at Willapa Bay, Washington,
north of the Columbia River, as second in command. There he
gained valuable leadership experience. Persson took charge of the
Gray's Harbor Station in 1922. Upon taking command, he had fifteen years experience in surf operations. By 1930, Hilman had lost
"track of how many missions he had been on . . . [and] how many
lives he had saved." The 36-foot motor lifeboats were, by this
time, more dependable. In May 1937, Hilman Persson would need
the use of a dependable motor lifeboat and all the knowledge he
had gained in thirty years of service.[53]

Friday, 7 May 1937 began much like any other day at the station. After morning colors at 8:00 A.M., the crew held drills until
9:00. The rest of the day they continued with the normal mun-
dane, day-to-day work around the station, such as mowing the
grass and equipment maintenance. To the south of Gray's Harbor,
in the Willapa Bay area, the American steam schooner *Trinidad,*
departed Raymond, Washington, with a load of lumber, bound for
San Francisco.[54]

Throughout the day, Persson, a careful observer of the
weather, noted the winds, which began light and from the
southeast, shifted to the south and steadily increased. By 8:00 P.M.,
the winds were howling at more than sixty miles per hour.
Meanwhile, the *Trinidad* had crossed the Willapa Bar and faced the
fury of the storm. The lumber schooner staggered "like a drunken
man" in the gale. For "several hours" the captain of the *Trinidad,*
Capt. I. Hellestone, battled the storm, but he then decided to put
back into Willapa Bay. *Trinidad* struck heavily on a shoal off the
north spit. The deckload of lumber broke loose and slammed into
the hull. The second mate, Werner Kraft, slipped and fell over the

side to his death. The crew of twenty, fearing for their lives, huddled on the bridge.[55]

Back at Gray's Harbor, Persson made an inspection of the station around 8:00 P.M. At 8:10, he received a telephone call from the Willapa Bay Station, known as the North Cove Station to locals. The watchstander in the lookout tower reported an unidentified steamer firing flares. Persson also learned from the watchstander that the Willapa Bay Station's lifeboat was already at sea after a fishing vessel in distress.[56]

The radio on board the Westport motor lifeboat could only receive messages. Persson ordered the Willapa Bay watchstander to call his boat every fifteen minutes with any news about the ship or Willapa Bay's motor lifeboat. Persson then reported the ship in distress to the district office and next put together a crew made up of Motor Mechanic Roy I. Anderson and Jesse W. Mathews, along with Surfmen Roy N. Woods and Daniel Hamaleinen. Hamaleinen, twenty-two, was the new man of the crew and had not yet been exposed to any "heavy weather work." Persson and his crew set out in their wooden 36-foot motor lifeboat.[57]

The motor lifeboat, despite the weather, had an "unexpectedly good passage over the bar." Persson noted a "strong northerly current running." Hilman told his crew to keep a sharp lookout for any signals from the *Trinidad* or the motor lifeboat sent from Willapa Bay Station, then went into the forward compartment to check for any messages. Much later, Hilman recalled that the small compartment was the "most uncomfortable place on the boat, with the bow diving and pounding into the sea and I did not want to subject any of the others to this torture." There was no news, and visibility "was fair."[58]

When Persson's motor lifeboat was about halfway to the entrance of Willapa Bay, the *Trinidad* fired another flare. Persson ordered one of his crewmen to fire a flare to show the ship's crew that help was on the way.[59] It took seven hours of battling the sea and current for the motor lifeboat to reach the north spit of Willapa Bay. The tide was low, and the lifeboat crossed the bar about two miles inside the bay. Hilman elected to cross the south spit, which he did not "think was breaking as hard as the bar." Halfway across, a large breaker hit the 36-footer, completely submerging the motor lifeboat and causing it to broach. Later, Persson would explain that when "you run on a break, a boat is like a car on ice and you lose control. The rudder, being in what I call loose water, has no affect on the boat and she will usually broach." Much later, Persson recalled, "I thought we were gone once. There was once we came within a hair's breath of capsizing." The seas drove the lifeboat back to the north spit again.[60]

As he got close to the distressed vessel, Persson spotted oil seeping from the *Trinidad*. Feeling that the oil might have some calming effect on the churning seas, Persson put his boat into the oily water and started in for the second try. "The stern was in the roughest water[,] so we came around the bow to her starboard side, where the water was comparatively calm," he would recall.[61] "Comparatively calm" is an old lifeboatman's understatement. A sailor on board the *Trinidad* saw it differently. "It didn't look like we would get away alive," he recalled. "Then just about daylight, the Coast Guard began working in. . . . I don't believe I ever lived a happier moment in my life than . . . when they came up under the lee side. Captain Persson was hanging on with one hand and waving directions with the other. The boat would rise up on a sea and then plunge down in the trough. . . . I was afraid sometimes they never would come up again[,] but the boat would bob up like a cork, and kept inching in closer."[62]

"There was danger in picking up lines in the wheel [propeller of the motor lifeboat] from the rigging hanging over her side," Persson remembered. "The bridge was still standing, with only one post holding up the port side. The crew was on the bridge, the only safe place on the ship, and when [we] came alongside they walked in orderly fashion to the starboard side and entered our boat. We were nearly level with the ship's deckload and at that time it was comparatively dry."[63] Again, the lifeboatman's "comparatively."

The sailor on board the *Trinidad*, however, recalled that "there was no smile on their faces . . . just set expressions . . . determination. They were taking an awful beating[,] too, their boat pitched and rolled and bounced like a rubber ball. To this hour I don't see how they made it. They would claw their way up to the 'Trinidad,' take off a couple of men and then the sea and wind would beat them away. They would haul around and pitch and roll their way back again and take off two or three more men. We almost prayed for them. They sure could take it and come back for more. And it wasn't only the sea[,] . . . there was rigging and gear plunging around, masts swaying, loading booms, lumber, and any minute that fore deckload was due to go . . . but they didn't pay much attention to it . . . which was plenty lucky for us."[64]

After taking off all the survivors, the heavy load of sailors made the motor lifeboat difficult to handle and "several times" Persson warned "the men to keep down close to the deck. At that, we took several breaks over the boat and when we got through, our faces were coated with oil."[65]

Once in sheltered waters, Persson contacted the oil screw vessel *Ruth E.* Afterward, the *Ruth E* took the survivors on board and transported them to Raymond. Persson put into Tokeland. A truck from the Gray's Harbor Station came to pick up the exhausted crew. Finally, the lifesavers returned to their station at 9:00 A.M., twelve and a half hours after setting out to rescue the crew of the *Trinidad*.[66] Hamaleinen, the surfman on his first heavy weather case, "performed like a veteran," Persson later remarked. "He's a doggone good man . . . and he didn't even get seasick."[67] The unknown sailor on board the *Trinidad* summed up what many survivors have felt when they saw a small U.S. Coast Guard boat heading toward them in almost impossible conditions: "Those guys got plenty of guts, take it from me. I'll praise them to my last day."[68]

For their work in rescuing twenty survivors from the *Trinidad*, Hilman J. Persson and his four-man crew received the Gold Life Saving Medal. Later, Persson would receive the Second Division Post, American Legion of Baltimore's Medal of Merit, an annual award for the most outstanding act of heroism in the United States.[69]

The U.S. Coast Guard transferred Hilman J. Persson in 1938 from Grays Harbor to District Headquarters in Seattle. Persson had a vacancy in the crew, so he had his son, Fridolph, sign papers to become a crewman. After Hillman was relieved of command, Fridolph enlisted on board the station, thus keeping the tradition of a Persson at the station since its commissioning. Fridolph served from 1938 to the end of World War II and then left the service. He later remembered that it "broke my Dad's heart."[70]

Hillman John Persson retired in 1939, while serving in the district office. He returned to active duty when the United States entered World War II and remained on duty until the end of the war. He died on 20 December 1973, at the age of eighty-four. "He came to the United States a young, naive boy," his son Fridolph said, "but became a loyal, patriotic American to the end of his life."[71]

SUBMARINE VERSUS MOTOR LIFEBOAT

During World War II, crews of the U.S. Coast Guard responded to two cases that again prove the determination and ingenuity of those serving at small boat stations. On 20 December 1941, less than two weeks after the Japanese attack on Pearl Harbor, Hawaii, the naval radio station at Humboldt Bay, along the northern California coast, received a message from the tanker *Emidio*. It was off the Blunt's Reef Lightship and needed assistance. After that terse message, the radio station received no further messages from the ship.[72]

A lookout at the Cape Mendocino Light Station, approximately thirty-eight miles south of the station, reported he had a tanker in view rounding the lightship but it did not appear in distress. Scant minutes later, the lightship, located four and a half miles from Cape Mendocino, reported the tanker proceeding northward. Other reports also tracked *Emidio* moving in a northerly direction with no apparent problems. The ship passed Humboldt Bay on a steady course and speed at 3:25 P.M. Thus far, having received only one distress message, no one could decide if the transmission was a hoax.

At 8:35 P.M., Warrant Officer Garner J. Churchill, command-ing officer of the Humboldt Bay lifeboat Station, received a mes-sage about *Emidio*. The tanker reported a Japanese torpedo attack near Blunt's Reef. The pilot of a naval patrol aircraft had seen *Emidio* "launch lifeboats" and an explosion at the stern of the ship. Afterward, the pilot had seen the wake of the torpedo and had dropped depth charges where he felt the submarine would lie, with no results. The pilot reported he had contact with the lifeboats and there were fifty-two men "in the water," with two men killed and one dying. What all the lookouts had observed was the *Emidio* proceeding northward without a crew on board.

The weather at Humboldt Bay turned foul. Rain squalls passed through the area, visibility ranged from zero to two hun-dred yards, and the bar was "very rough." Added to this danger-ous mix, fear of a Japanese invasion caused the darkening of all lighted aids to navigation. The largest U.S. Coast Guard cutter available to help was the *Shawnee*, a 158-foot oceangoing tug. His long years of experience in northern California waters made Churchill notify his command that if the *Shawnee* could not cross the bar, he was ready with his 36-foot motor lifeboat.

There could not have been a better commanding officer than Churchill at a station on this terrible night. Churchill had enlisted in the U.S. Coast Guard in 1924 at San Francisco, serving his first duty at Humboldt Bay before transferring to the Fort Point lifeboat Station at San Francisco. He then returned to Humboldt Bay and served there until he retired in 1954. A measure of the man can be found in the 1939 case of the yacht *Reta*, which capsized on the Humboldt bar. Churchill and his 36-foot motor lifeboat crew rescued four people from the yacht. The U.S. Coast Guard planned to award Churchill a Gold Life Saving Medal for the rescue, but his crew was to receive the Silver Medal. Churchill refused the Gold Medal, saying that "he had done no more than his men." In the end, Churchill and the entire boat crew received the Silver Life Saving Medal. Churchill received a promotion to warrant officer on 15 February 1938.[73] By 20 December 1941, Churchill had amassed seventeen years of U.S. Coast Guard experience working with lifeboats, including at least sixteen years at Humboldt Bay.

A decision not to send the *Shawnee* did not deter Churchill. He selected a crew of four U.S. Coast Guardsmen—Boatswain's Mate 1st Class Clifford J. Hall, Motor Machinist 1st Class Thomas E. Jackson, Seaman 1st Class Paul R. Chance, and Seaman 2d Class Robert J. Weaver—to accompany him in the 36-foot motor lifeboat. Churchill had a message passed to the army not to fire on the small boat. This was a wise move, as the West Coast continued to live in fear of an invasion by the Japanese and gun crews tended to fire at anything they did not recognize. On a stormy night, an unidentified boat might just let loose a hail of deadly fire.[74]

Churchill, with no lighted aids to navigation to help him, approached the dark bar. There the crew faced "heavy swells and occasional sluffers [breaking waves] running." A breaking wave on a bar is one of the most dangerous conditions a mariner can face. As oceanographer William G. Van Doren notes, "Under extreme conditions, pressures in excess of one ton per square foot have been measured in breaking waves, while wind [wave] pressures rarely exceed 10 to 12 pounds per square foot."[75]

By 1:05 A.M. on 21 December, Churchill and his crew of four were across the bar heading southwest at approximately eight knots. Two hours later, the bow lookout reported an "unlighted object" off the port bow. Churchill made a slow, cautious approach to the unidentified object. At a range of one hundred yards, the lifeboat's crew could make out the dim outline of some type of surface vessel. It was without masts, stack, or deck housing, dead in the water, with its bow pointed north.

Churchill attempted to signal the vessel with a signal light. The weather conditions caused the light from the signal lamp to hamper the U.S. Coast Guardsmen's night vision. No return signal came from the mystery ship. Taking a prudent course of action, Churchill slowly turned the 36-footer away from the vessel. After this maneuver, the unknown contact began making headway. The wary Coast Guardsmen realized the vessel was now tracking them.

Churchill pushed the throttle forward on the motor lifeboat. The still-unidentified vessel closed rapidly.

At fifty yards, it "became evident" that the vessel intended to ram the lifeboat. Churchill waited until a large Pacific swell began to lift the 36-footer then added more throttle and laid the wheel hard right. The seas made the maneuver so fast and sharp the vessel could not follow and it went off to the southeast. Churchill then ran for a few minutes, hove to, and shut down his engine. The mystery ship continued to search the area for the lifeboat. As the tracking vessel rose on a swell, it was "silhouetted against the reflected glow of lights from the city of Eureka to the [northeast]." The U.S. Coast Guardsmen now knew they were dealing with a Japanese submarine.

Shortly after 4:00 A.M., the submarine disappeared. Undaunted, Churchill continued with his mission. About forty-five minutes later, the lifeboat crew spotted *Emidio*. Churchill circled the tanker. Using the boat's searchlight, the U.S. Coast Guardsmen could see no sign of life on board the ship. Furthermore, all the ship's lifeboats were missing from their davits.

At 8:00 A.M. a Navy PBY patrol aircraft arrived on scene and flew around *Emidio*. Churchill could not contact the aircraft and, at 9:30, decided to depart the tanker and return to Humboldt Bay. Churchill and the aircraft crew did not know that the survivors from the tanker were on Blunt's Reef Lightship.[76]

The return to the lifeboat station began slowly because the heavy seas threw "walls of water on board." About four miles southeast of *Emidio*'s position, a lookout on board the motor lifeboat spotted a periscope six hundred yards off their starboard beam. The periscope disappeared. Churchill changed course. Fifteen minutes later, another lookout spotted the periscope again, this time at least six hundred yards away and abaft the starboard beam. The crew of the motor lifeboat was able to observe the submarine tracking them because the captain of the sub kept his periscope above the surface for at least five minutes at a time before lowering it and disappearing.

Churchill and his weary, cold crew returned to their station at 12:35 P.M. Some legends have it that Churchill tried to lure the submerged submarine into shallow waters, hoping to damage it. If true, one wonders if Churchill, had he been successful, would have painted a silhouette of a submarine on his 36-foot motor lifeboat. That would have turned the head of any veteran of convoy duty.

Emidio eventually broke up on the rocks off Crescent City, California, approximately eighty-seven miles to the north of the Humboldt Bay Station. A section of the bow still remains near the beach in Crescent City.[77] There is no monument to Garner J. Churchill and his crew, who, on a SAR case, came face to face with a different sort of danger.[78]

RESCUE BY SHOESTRING

On the night of 31 March 1943, the Soviet freighter *Lamut* battled its way through a typical Pacific Northwest storm. Blowing spray and gale-whipped rain cut visibility, and seas built higher and higher. *Lamut*'s captain lost his bearings and the freighter struck hard on the rocks of Teahwhit Head, approximately seventy miles south of the Strait of Juan de Fuca on Washington's north coast. Even today, as a part of Olympic National Park, the area remains a wild, rocky coastline. *Lamut* came to rest in a rough U-shaped headland, with almost sheer cliffs on two sides, the tallest 270 feet high. Under the relentless pounding of the seas, the ship heeled onto its port beam. The captain realized the danger of launching a lifeboat in this location but felt he had no other course of action if he wanted to save any of his crew of fifty-two. The lowering of the boat turned into a disaster. One of the boat falls snapped, critically injuring a nineteen-year-old woman crewmember and hurling another woman to her death in the raging seas. With the port lifeboat gone, the crew would soon be lost if help did not come from another source.[79]

The 6:00 A.M. to noon patrol from the U.S. Coast Guard beach patrol station at LaPush, about five miles north of the wreck site, noticed debris along the shoreline. Then the beach patrol came upon the body of the Soviet woman. Two teams of U.S. Coast Guardsmen from LaPush and the nearby Quillayute River Station immediately began to search for the wreck. One group took the station's small boat and started to search southward. The boat crew located the *Lamut,* but the seas and the location of the ship made it impossible for them to help.[80]

Another search party of twelve U.S. Coast Guardsmen had driven close to where they thought the ship might lie. Grabbing axes and ropes, they began to push through the forest to reach the beach. They had to hack through a lush, temperate rain forest not unlike a jungle. Many years later, Mike James, at the time an eighteen-year-old U.S. Coast Guardsman, recalled that it took at least two hours to make the mile to the beach.[81]

The search party came out about two miles away from the shipwreck. Nearing the wreck site, they found the way blocked by a high, rocky cliff. Now the U.S. Coast Guardsmen had to employ rock-climbing skills. First they worked their way up the steep cliff, then they had to traverse a narrow ridge. Contemporary photographs of the actual rescue attempt are dramatic. The U.S. Coast Guardsmen inched their way across the rain-slick rocks with the wind tugging at them. Finally, the twelve men reached a spot directly above *Lamut.* More than two hundred feet below, the Soviet sailors were clinging to the dangerously slanted deck. A scrawled sign proclaimed "1 wuman ill." The Coast Guardsmen knew additional help was on the way, but time was running out. The twelve, even with their limited resources, decided to attempt to get the crew off *Lamut.*[82]

The rescuers weighted the end of a line with a rock and heaved it to the stricken sailors. It fell short by inches. Again and again they tried. Many years later, James recalled that one of the rescuers, a Coast Guardsman from Pennsylvania, Joe Mufasanti, hit upon a solution that remains unique in the annals of U.S. Coast Guard rescues. He suggested that everyone on the ridge remove his shoelaces, tie them together, and add this to the rope. Feeling they had nothing to lose, the men followed Mufasanti's idea. One man then "stood precariously on the edge of the cliff" and heaved the line. It reached! Quickly, the Soviet seamen tied on a heavier line, which the U.S. Coast Guardsmen pulled across. A series of heavier and heavier lines passed between the ridge and the ship. At last, a strong hawser stretched between *Lamut* and the rocks.[83]

The Soviets now faced the ordeal of going hand over hand along the hawser to the rocks. Slowly pulling their way across, with the "snarling, crashing breakers below," *Lamut*'s crew knew that a "slip would have meant instant death." Later, some Soviet sailors "admitted that fear alone impelled them onward."[84] The hawser sagged under the weight of the sailors, and the Soviets reached an undercut cave ledge about halfway up the cliff. *Lamut*'s crew rigged a stretcher for the injured woman. Quickly the rig passed along the hawser to the cave.

Next, the rescuers rigged their line to the sailors on the lower ledge. *Lamut*'s sailors then worked their way up to the ridge. The woman in the stretcher proved the most difficult to get up the cliff, but one by one the Soviets struggled up the rock face. U.S. Coast Guardsmen helped *Lamut*'s crew along the narrow ridge and down the cliff on the land side. The official report noted that the "journey down . . . was as difficult as the climb up the seaward side had been."[85]

"Showing the effects of the terrific ordeal," the Soviets trudged in groups along the beach. They reached the trail hacked out by the U.S. Coast Guardsmen and then trudged out to the road and waiting trucks. Darkness was falling when "the last of the crew staggered from the swampy trail, coated with mud and sodden with fatigue."[86]

Forty-five years after the event, when questioned whether he thought it might be impossible to rescue the Soviets, Mike James responded, "Never gave it a [thought]: *Semper Paratus.*"[87]

8 | The Rescue of *Pendelton*

On Monday, 18 February 1952, the U.S. Coast Guard faced the unthinkable along the Massachusetts coast. Two tankers, *Fort Mercer* and *Pendelton,* within forty miles of each other, battling high winds and seas, broke in two off Cape Cod. Cutters and motor lifeboats, supported by aircraft, eventually rescued seventy of the eighty-four sailors marooned on the four sinking sections of ships.[1] Thirty-two of the survivors came from the tanker *Pendelton,* and all owed their lives to the bravery of a 36-foot motor lifeboat crew from a lifeboat station in Chatham, Massachusetts.

The 503-foot 10,448-ton tanker *Pendelton* departed Baton Rouge, Louisiana, on Tuesday, 12 February 1952.[2] Under the command of Capt. John Fitzgerald, it carried kerosene and heating oil and shipped a crew of forty. Captain Fitzgerald shaped a course for Boston. Late on Sunday, 17 February, the tanker arrived off the approach to Boston. Fitzgerald found himself in very foul weather and wisely opted to stand off. He ordered *Pendelton* into Massachusetts Bay at slow speed. The weather deteriorated. Fitzgerald now faced a severe New England nor'easter.

By 4:00 A.M. on Monday, the eighteenth, water was washing over the stern of *Pendelton,* but the tanker continued to ride "nicely." Spray from the heavy seas, mixed with snow, further lowered visibility. *Pendelton* slowly rounded the tip of Cape Cod off Provincetown, and Captain Fitzgerald shaped a more southerly course.[3]

At approximately 5:50 A.M., sailors on board the tanker heard a series of explosive noises. Shortly after that, *Pendelton* broke in two. The bow, with Captain Fitzgerald and seven crewmen on board it, drifted off. Machinery in the stern section continued to operate, providing lights for the remainder of the crew in that section. Chief Engineer Raymond Sybert took charge and mustered the thirty-two survivors now under his charge.

In seas estimated at sixty feet by nearby U.S. Coast Guard cutters, *Pendelton*'s bow section drifted southward toward deep water. The stern also drifted southerly, but about six miles off Cape Cod. No one on *Pendelton* had time to get off a distress call.[4]

By midmorning of Monday, the U.S. Coast Guard lifeboat station at Chatham, Massachusetts, had received word that a ship, *Fort Mercer,* had broken in two. At the same time, the station watchstander was receiving telephone calls from local fishermen to help them as their boats broke their moorings in the harbor.[5]

Warrant Officer Daniel W. Cluff, commanding officer of the Chatham Lifeboat Station, received orders from the First Coast Guard District Headquarters in Boston to send a 36-foot motor lifeboat out to *Fort Mercer.* Boatswain's Mate 1st Class Bernard C. Webber overheard the orders. He wondered about the chances of a small lifeboat finding the "ship amid the blinding snow and raging seas with only a compass to guide them." Even if the crew did not freeze, Webber thought, it was unlikely the men could launch in such weather.[6]

Cluff, nevertheless, ordered Chief Boatswain's Mate Donald Bangs to select a crew and get underway in the CG-36383. Bangs detailed Engineman 1st Class Emory H. Hayes, Boatswain's Mate

3d Class (Provisional) Antonio F. Ballerini, and Seaman Richard J. Ciccone as his crew then started for the motor lifeboat.[7]

Warrant Officer Cluff ordered Webber to select a crew and take the CG-36500, at nearby Old Harbor, to help secure the adrift fishing vessels. Webber and his crew worked most of the morning in heavy snow and wind. By the time they secured the vessels, they were "very cold and tired."

Upon his return to the station, Webber received a call to report to Cluff. The exhausted Webber learned there were now two ships broken in two. Reports indicated the other ship, later identified as *Pendelton,* adrift with part of it close to the beach somewhere between the towns of Chatham and Orleans and near Nauset Beach. Cluff ordered Webber to take his crew in a four-wheel-drive truck and meet with the Nauset Lifeboat Station to check out the sighting.

The two crews met and made their way out to Nauset Beach. A break in the heavy weather revealed "half of a ship, black and sinister," wallowing in the heavy seas, "frothing each time" it hit a swell. Webber estimated the aft section on a course toward Chatham. There was no way for the two U.S. Coast Guard crews to communicate with the Chatham Station; Webber leaped into his truck and drove to the station to sound the alarm. The U.S. Coast Guardsmen arrived back at the Chatham lifeboat Station at 5:30 P.M. in near darkness. An experimental radar at the unit located two targets: the bow section of *Pendelton* drifting out to sea and the stern wallowing near the beach. Chief Bangs and his crew on board the other 36-foot motor lifeboat continued their battle to reach the bow section. Bangs finally reached the bow. Seeing no signs of life, he started toward shore. Another ship radioed that they saw someone on the bow; Bangs received orders to return to the bow section.[8]

Warrant Officer Cluff realized he had to send another boat into this terrible night. He turned to Webber and told him to select a crew and take the CG-36500 out across the bar to the stern section of *Pendelton.*

Webber was twenty-four years old and eight days short of six years in U.S. Coast Guard. Years later, he recalled that he had agreed with Cluff's decision. After all, he knew the "waters and territory" better than anyone else at the station. Webber had no illusions of what awaited him out there in the darkness. "A sinking feeling came over me," he later admitted. "I thought about many things before answering [Cluff]." Webber then replied, "Yes, Sir, Mr. Cluff, I'll get ready." Engineman Second Class Andrew J. Fitzgerald, Seaman Richard P. Livesey, and Seaman Erving E. Maske, a crewmember of the Stonehorse Lightship who was at the station waiting for the weather to clear to return to his lightship, made up Webber's crew.[9]

Webber and his crew drove to a wharf at the Chatham fish pier. They rowed out in the darkness in a dory to reach the CG-36500's moorings. An experienced fisherman called out, "You guys better get lost before you get too far out." In other words, stall and do not go out. Such a comment from an old salt increased Webber's anxiety. Nevertheless, the four U.S. Coast Guardsmen boarded the motor lifeboat and started at 5:55 P.M. from Old Harbor into the teeth of the storm.

The ninety-horsepower gas engine of the CG-36500, not yet fully warm, sputtered as the motor lifeboat drew closer to the bar. Even above the wind and the motor lifeboat's engine, the crew heard the roar of the ocean. Already drenched and cold, the motor lifeboat crew had yet to cross the bar. Webber felt if he turned back, no one would complain. His crew suddenly broke out into "songs like *Rock of Ages* and *Harbor Lights*." Asked about it later, Webber could not explain this outburst.

Webber radioed the station. Was there any change of orders? Cluff's orders: continue out to sea. The single-propeller motor lifeboat approached the bar. Webber radioed the station again and again received instructions to continue out to sea. "At that point a shiver went through me," he recalled. "Questions came into my mind. Where would we go? With only a magnetic compass to navigate by, no radar to assist us in locating a broken ship in the blackness of a night full of sleet, snow and raging seas, how could we possibly do it?" Webber realized that his profession was "the sea and to save those in peril upon it."

After warning his crew to hang on, Webber advanced the boat's throttle. "Fortunately, I really couldn't see the conditions ahead," he remembered. "I wasn't aware of what was about to happen, otherwise I might have turned around right there and then and headed back in."

The first wave threw the 20,170-pound motor lifeboat into the air. It landed in the trough of the waves. Another wave struck the 36-footer, and water cascaded down upon it. The windshield broke. Frigid sea water rushed through the broken windshield, knocking Webber to the deck of the coxswain's platform. The compass was carried away. Webber grabbed the steering wheel and fought to keep the bow into the seas.

Another large wave laid the motor lifeboat on its beam. The engine stopped. Extreme rolling caused the engine to lose its gasoline prime. Engineman Fitzgerald fought to open the hatch leading into the engine compartment. Inside the small, foul-smelling space, Fitzgerald managed to restart the engine. The sea threw Fitzgerald around the compartment, bruising and burning him. Each time the engine cut off, the engineer bravely reentered the compartment.[10]

The waves changed; they were farther apart. Webber realized this meant the motor lifeboat had crossed the bar into deeper water. Deeper water meant only relative safety. Webber and his crew now faced seas estimated as high as a six-story building. Up a steep wave the 36-footer toiled. Plunging over the crest, the lifeboat surfed down the backside. Webber reversed the engine to keep from burying the bow into the next wave. Again and again this continued. Maske recalled, "You would ride the top of one wave and hit the bottom on the next. Another wave would come and then we'd pray."[11]

Years later, Webber recalled he had no idea of their position. There was no radio communication. The four U.S. Coast Guardsmen, pumped with adrenalin, cold and wet, continued to hang onto the motor lifeboat. Webber now felt the weather turning worse, if that were possible. The crew continued their battle.

Webber, feeling alone and forgotten, knew he had ten to twelve hours before sunrise. Again he feared for their safety.[12]

Suddenly, a dark shape loomed in front of them. Webber sent a crewman forward to turn on the motor lifeboat's searchlight. Caught in the beam of light was a huge tunnel of broken and twisted steel. Against all odds, the crew of the CG-36500 had come upon the stern of *Pendelton*. Webber maneuvered his motor lifeboat along the port side of the stern section. Spotting no signs of life, he thought everyone on board had perished and his crew's long fight with the sea had been for naught. Rounding the stern of *Pendelton,* lights appeared on the wreck. Webber spotted a crewman high on the ship frantically waving his arms. The figure disappeared, only to reappear with a line of sailors along the rail. Sailors shouted down to the lifeboat, but Webber could only catch snatches over the wind and the seas. After their long battle with the sea, Webber thought the sailors on board *Pendelton* might be safer on the stern of their ship. *Pendelton*'s sailors thought differently. A sailor put a rope ladder over the side. *Pendelton*'s crew started down the ladder.

A stunned Webber thought, "Good Lord, they are coming over the side and want us to pick them off the ladder!" The first sailor reached the bottom of the rope ladder and found himself dunked into the sea each time the hulk wallowed in the heavy seas.

Webber's crewmen made their way toward the bow of the 36-footer. They knew the dangers facing them. Added to the difficulties of maintaining their footing and a precarious handhold on a pitching, rolling motor lifeboat, the three crewmen somehow had to steady the sailors leaping onto the bow of the motor lifeboat.

Webber started toward the rope ladder. He timed the actions of the sea. The sailor lowest on the ladder leaped to the motor lifeboat and landed hard on the boat. The lifesavers on the bow grabbed the sailor and helped him down into the forward survivor's compartment. Webber backed away. He again repeated his approach.[13] The other sailors clung to the rope ladder. The men on the ladder swung away from the ship as the hulk laid over, then slammed into the hull as it rolled the other way. Despite the beating, *Pendelton*'s sailors clung to the ladder, knowing this was their only way to safety.

Twenty times Webber brought the 36-foot motor lifeboat alongside the hulk of *Pendelton*. Later, in typical lifeboatman's laconic understatement, he recalled the small motor lifeboat "getting crowded." The large number of rescued sailors made the craft heavier and harder to handle. Webber wondered whether he should stop. Recognizing *Pendelton*'s sailors were now "frantic" to get off the hulk, he decided to continue. Extreme fear gripped the sailors on the ladder. Some leaped too soon. At least five missed the motor lifeboat and plunged into the cold, churning sea. Through "super-human strength" Webber's crewmen pulled them on board. Maske recalled that Fitzgerald and Livesey were on the 36-footer's bow. "They held on with one hand to anything they could grab and fished sailors out of the water . . . with the other hand[,] grabbing on to whatever they could—belts, pants, jackets."[14]

Webber again thought about leaving the remaining men on board the stern of *Pendelton* but decided he could not. Finally, in what seemed like an eternity, only one man remained grasping the rope ladder. George "Tiny" Myers weighed at least three hundred pounds. Myers throughout the ordeal had helped others to the ladder before thinking of himself. Now it was his turn. Webber again maneuvered the motor lifeboat to the stern of *Pendelton*. By now the craft handled sluggishly. The bow of the lifeboat approached the ladder. Myers leaped too soon. He plunged into the sea. Webber backed down hard. His crewmen scanned the seas with the searchlight and spotted Myers under the "very stern" of *Pendelton*, clinging desperately to a blade of the stopped ship's propeller.

Again Webber made the difficult approach to the hulk. This time he had to "stick the bow of the lifeboat directly toward" Myers to get close enough to "grab ahold of him." As Webber started in, a large sea picked up the heavily laden lifeboat and flung it toward *Pendelton*. Webber backed down hard but to no avail. He later recalled that he saw "the fright on [Tiny's] face" just before the motor lifeboat slammed into *Pendelton*, pinning Myers between it and the lifeboat. Another large wave washed the 36-

footer way from the hulk and the dead Myers. The stern of
Pendelton rose up and rolled over.

With the roll-over of the stern section, darkness surrounded
Webber's crew and the thirty-two survivors. Thirty-six sailors and
U.S. Coast Guardsmen now huddled in the forward survivors compartment, the engine compartment and coxswain flat. Webber had
no idea of his position, other than somewhere off Chatham. The
radios in a 36-footer seldom functioned correctly in bad weather,
just when you needed them. On this night, with many other units
involved, the airways crackled with static and voices. Webber
decided he must try to give a status report. He pressed the transmit button on the radio telephone's handset. Webber reported
"thirty-two survivors and four crewmen on board." The radio
worked! It worked too well. A steady stream of instructions bom-
barded Webber from every U.S. Coast Guard cutter and shore unit,
telling him to bring the survivors to them. Everyone wanted to
micromanage the situation. Webber heard "arguments going on
between units as to what we should do, and in typical government
service fashion, who was responsible for what and who outranked
whom." He reached over and turned off the radio.[15]

The young coxswain briefed the survivors and his crew that
he intended to head the motor lifeboat toward land and ground it
on the nearest sheltered beach. Once the 36-footer grounded, he
would hold it there with the engine and the survivors could leap
into the shallow water. All on board agreed with his plan, and the
boat started toward the beach.

More than fifty years after the rescue, crewman Richard P.
Livesey recalled that on the run to the beach, the following waves
broke over them constantly: "I was standing in the well deck
[between the bow survivor's compartment and the engine com-
partment] with my back to the radio antenna [attached to forward
survivor's compartment]. I don't know how many sailors were
around me. We were jammed in like a pack of sardines. I was having a bad time breathing, the water was up to my chest and a lot
of times over my head. I just prayed Webber would be able to get
us back over the bar."[16]

As fate would have it, Webber managed to bring the motor lifeboat to the buoy marking the entrance to Old Harbor at Chatham. Once more he turned on the radio and gave his position, along with a request for assistance at the fish pier. Again the radio again crackled with overdirection, and again Webber snapped it off.[17]

Webber maneuvered the CG-36500 to the pier, where many men, women, and children waited to help the survivors. As *Pendelton*'s sailors departed, Webber recalled, "I began to tremble and sob. With my crewman, [Erving] Maske, beside me I unashamedly cried in the near solitude and gave thanks to God for guiding us through the unknown."

For their amazing rescue, Bernard C. Webber, Andrew J. Fitzgerald, Richard P. Livesey, and Erving E. Maske received the Gold Life Saving Medal.[18] Webber recalled that in "those days there was no consideration of the trauma personnel experienced."[19] George G. "Tiny" Myers remains etched in the memories of Bernard C. Webber and Richard Livesey.[20] More than half a century after his amazing feat, Webber remarked, "My killing [Myers] with the lifeboat left an everlasting mark. . . . I can still see the expression on his face and the look in his eyes just before it happened. Not a day has gone by . . . that I haven't relived the whole deal."[21]

9 | I Thought It Was the End

In 1961, the U.S. Coast Guard lifeboat station at Cape Disappointment, Washington, responded to a call considered by many "routine." Old salts in the maritime search and rescue business usually insist, however, that there is no such thing as routine, for anything can happen when a rescue boat puts out to sea.

For those in the U.S. Coast Guard's small boat community, the Pacific Northwest has a reputation for high surf. One location in particular has a fearsome reputation: the mouth of the Columbia River, known to mariners as the "Graveyard of the Pacific." The Columbia Maritime Museum in Astoria, Oregon, estimates that two thousand ships and craft, two hundred of them major cases, have been lost in the area over the years.[1] It sometimes appears the question is not whether someone will die in a given year, but how many will die. High waves of the Pacific Ocean meeting the power of the Columbia River, combined with a bar near the mouth of the river, make this an area of consistently treacherous waves. This fact of nature caused the U.S. Coast Guard to establish a heavy weather school nearby to teach coxswains how to handle motor lifeboats in high, rough seas.

At the mouth of the Columbia River, some two miles in width, sits Cape Disappointment, Washington, to the north and Clatsop Spit, Oregon, to the south. Near Clatsop Spit is an area of high surf known to U.S. Coast Guardsmen in the area as "Death Row." Hard to the west of Cape Disappointment, and just north of the northern buoy line, lies the treacherous Peacock Spit. On 18 July 1841, it sank the *Peacock,* a ship of the U.S. Exploring Expedition commanded by Lt. Charles Wilkes, U.S. Navy. The 559-ton sloop of war had survived travels in the North and South Atlantic, the Antarctic, South Pacific, and parts of the North Pacific, but not the Columbia River.[2]

The mouth of the Columbia stretches between a south jetty extending two and a half miles due west of Clatsop Spit and the north jetty, which runs parallel to but slightly south of Peacock Spit. The main approach to the river is wedge shaped, two miles at the mouth and half a mile at the river entrance proper. Along the north of the channel, the left-hand side, a line of buoys stretched, numbered 1, 3, 5, 7, and 9. The color of these buoys in 1961 was black, and people on the river referred to the buoys on this side of the channel as the "black line." Along the south of the channel, the right-hand side, buoys with numbers 2, 4, 6, and 8 formed the "red line." The most shallow location in the channel, known as "the bar," extends between buoys 4 and 8 and 5 and 9. In heavy weather, swells first start to break on Clatsop Spit between the south jetty and on Peacock Spit, just north of the north jetty. As conditions worsen, waves can break completely across the channel. Breaking waves on a bar is one of the worse conditions confronting a mariner. Such waves exert more pressure than wind-driven swells. Normally, when the bar is rough, the safest passage is on the northern side of the channel.[3] The currents in the channel, however, "are not always predictable." A "strong northerly or northwesterly set [movement of current] occurs from the black buoy lines between buoys 1 and 7," often forcing a vessel onto Peacock Spit.

In 1961, the U.S. Coast Guard had two lifeboat stations guarding the river. On the north side, and closest to the mouth,

Cape Disappointment Lifeboat Station had two 40-foot utility boats and one 36-foot motor lifeboat, and a station complement of fifteen. On the south, the Oregon side, Point Adams Lifeboat Station had a 52-foot motor lifeboat, two 36-foot motor lifeboats, and two 40-foot utility boats, with a station complement of twenty-one.[4]

The Columbia River area in 1961 supported a large commercial and sport fishery. Commercial crabbing usually started in December, just when consistently bad weather and high seas began. It was during this time that the lifeboat stations dealt with some of their most difficult rescues (this is still the case today at Cape Disappointment).

At 4:15 P.M. on Thursday, 12 January 1961, Roy Gunnari, the master of the fishing vessel *Jana Jo,* radioed the Cape Disappointment Station, near Ilwaco, Washington, and informed the radio watchstander of a fishing vessel in distress. Gunnari said that the skipper of *Mermaid,* a 34-foot fishing vessel of twelve gross tons, had talked to him on a secondary radio frequency via the marine operator. The skipper relayed that his vessel had lost its rudder above buoy 14, was drifting toward treacherous Peacock Spit, and needed immediate assistance.[5]

The watchstander called the senior petty officer (noncommissioned officer) on board the Cape Disappointment Station, Boatswain's Mate 1st Class Darrell J. Murray. Murray's officer in charge, Chief Boatswain's Mate Doyle S. Porter, was absent at the Ilwaco hospital, where his wife had just given birth to his son. Murray, a boatswain's mate with "long experience" at lifeboat stations, immediately checked the weather.[6] The wind near the mouth of the Columbia River was south to southwest at thirty-five to forty knots, with westerly swells on the bar at eight to fifteen feet and breaking seas on Clatsop and Peacock Spits. Visibility ranged from six to eight miles in rain squalls, with fog banks lingering on the horizon. The National Weather Service's morning forecast called for small craft warnings. Fishing vessels and deep draft ships, under pilotage, continued to cross the bar.

Murray decided to send a 40-foot utility boat, the CG-40564, and a 36-foot motor lifeboat, the CG-36454, to the scene. The 40-footer was a fast boat, but normally it worked in sheltered waters. Murray knew speed was essential: a rudderless fishing vessel drifting into breaking waves upon Peacock Spit faced great danger. By Columbia River standards, the weather was not that threatening, so Murray opted for the 40-footer's speed. This would allow the boat to reach the *Mermaid* quickly and get a line on the fishing vessel before it drifted into deadly Peacock Spit. Murray ordered the slower 36-foot motor lifeboat as backup. Murray detailed Engineman 2d Class Terrance A. Lowe and Seaman Acie B. Maxwell as his crew on board the 40-footer and directed Seaman Boatswain Larry B. Edwards to take charge of the 36-footer, with Fireman Brian H. Johnson and Seaman Apprentice James L. Croker as crewmen. Edwards, although not a petty officer, had passed his examinations for boatswain's mate and was close to being promoted. He had worked as a coxswain for the last five months, causing Chief Porter to judge him a "competent" boat handler and familiar with the Columbia River bar.

Murray, as coxswain, and his crew quickly boarded the 40-footer and got underway out into the river. He established communications with the station and *Jana Jo*. The owner of *Mermaid*, Bert E. Bergman, continued to transmit on a secondary frequency, which slowed the relayed information to Murray. Murray checked via radio with the lookout tower watchstander, who reported his failure to spot *Mermaid*. Arriving on scene, Murray could not locate *Mermaid*. He decided to take station near buoy 9 and await the arrival of the slower 36-footer, then change boats and proceed across the bar. Chief Porter, meanwhile, arrived at the station and immediately went to the lookout tower.

At just this time, the lookout tower watch spotted a boat in Peacock Spit. Years later, Murray recalled that this caused everything to "turn from somnambulant to [adrenalin] alert."[7] There remained approximately two hours of daylight. The forecast called for canceling the weather warnings by 5:00 P.M., the tide was on the last ebb, and it seemed the "optimum bar crossing time."[8] After discussing the changed circumstances with his officer in charge, Chief Porter, via radio, and with his crew, Murray took the 40-footer across the bar.

Once around the north jetty, Murray and his crew spotted a vessel "in about the 3rd line of surf" in Peacock Spit.[9] He maneuvered through the surf, trying to get close to the boat. The 40-footer ran into a large swell that stood it on its stern. As the senior petty officer righted his boat, a radio call from *Jana Jo* identified the boat in Peacock Spit as *Mermaid*. Murray radioed *Jana Jo* to meet outside the surf zone. The marine operator then radioed that she had *Mermaid* on her frequency. This allowed Murray to have his first actual communications with *Mermaid*. He next requested the fishing vessel's skipper to shine a light on the low clouds. Murray spotted the signal and made for the location, just as the weather started to worsen.

As Murray and his crew approached the location of *Mermaid*, they discussed "what might happen if they [the *Mermaid*] just drifted into the beach, could they survive it?"[10] The two people on board *Mermaid* settled this question by waving and calling for help. Within "15 minutes" Murray and his crew had taken the fishing vessel in tow.[11] Safely outside the surf zone, the rescue crew brought *Mermaid* alongside the 40-footer. The senior U.S. Coast Guardsman discussed with Bergman that Murray felt they had two options. One, take *Mermaid* farther offshore, then put both fishermen on the 40-footer, turn the vessel loose, and make for the Columbia River Lightship. The other option consisted of towing the fishing vessel out to the lightship. The latter had many things against it. Rudderless, *Mermaid* needed something to keep it in line with the 40-footer. Normally a drogue, a sea anchor, would accomplish this task. An earlier high-level U.S. Coast Guard decision, however, had removed drogues from the boat, which left the 40-footer crew without a sea anchor to pass to the fishing vessel. *Mermaid*'s crew tried buckets, but this did not work. Murray suggested that Bergman tie two or three crab pots together and stream them behind *Mermaid*. This worked. Although this action solved the problem of towing, it restricted the tow to no speed "beyond barely making headway." Bergman remained "adamant" about not leaving his vessel. This left the final plan of towing the fishing vessel to buoy 1 and await help.[12]

Back at Cape Disappointment Station, Chief Porter monitored the events from the lookout tower. The lookout tower, perched on a high bluff, commands a sweeping view of the mouth of the Columbia River. Chief Porter contacted Murray by radio and discussed the situation. Although not unduly alarmed, the chief decided that darkness and the worsening weather could make this rescue difficult. He ordered Murray to tow *Mermaid* to the entrance buoy and heave to, with the 36-footer standing by. Porter also called the Point Adams Station, located across the river in Oregon, and requested their 52-foot wooden motor lifeboat, the *Triumph*, start toward the scene and take over the tow. Next, Porter reported the developing case to his group commander and Thirteenth Coast Guard District Rescue Coordination Center (RCC) in Seattle. Thus far, almost everyone in the chain of command had treated this as a "routine" case.

On board the 36-footer, Seaman Edwards struggled to locate the 40-footer and *Mermaid*. The radio reception on board the 36-footer was weak and full of static. On the outbound leg, the motor lifeboat ran into heavy swells and green water, which pounded the twenty-two-year-old wooden boat. Considerable spray forced Edwards to lower the spray shield and windows for better visibility. He finally located the 40-footer, with *Mermaid* in tow, and escorted them to buoy number 1. Seaman Edwards then noticed that his radio antenna was broken. Worse, a check of the stern compartment revealed seawater in it. He promptly ordered his crewmen to keep checking the compartment and radioed the condition of his boat to the station.

Across the river at the Point Adams Lifeboat Station, scheduled for coxswain duty on board the motor lifeboat, was Boatswain's Mate 1st Class Willis P. Miller. Boatswain's Mate 1st Class John C. Culp, however, volunteered to take the *Triumph* out if something should happen while Miller went "home for a few minutes to allow his wife to go to the store." Thirty years later,

Joan Miller remembered her husband saying, "Hurry up, I have a call," as she returned home.[13]

While Miller was at home, Senior Chief Boatswain's Mate Warren C. Berto, the officer in charge of the Point Adams Station, received the call for assistance from Cape Disappointment. He ordered the 52-foot motor lifeboat *Triumph* out to buoy number 1 to relieve Murray of his tow. Culp, thirty-one, with two years of operations on the Columbia River, was a veteran lifeboatman in these waters. Three other veterans and two "relatively" new men made up Culp's crew. One of the new men, Engineman 3d Class Gordon E. Huggins, twenty-two, had reported to the Point Adams Station on 9 November 1960. Huggins, like Culp, did not have duty on board the *Triumph* this night but asked if he could "take [the engineer's] place so I could get trained on the boat."[14]

Culp shoved off at 5:05 P.M., five minutes after receiving the request from the Cape Disappointment Station. The lowering weather and increasing seas en route caused the nine-mile trip to the Cape Disappointment boats and *Mermaid* to take just over two hours. Years later, Huggins recalled that at about "bouy 8 seas were 25 to 30 feet. Culp had everyone put on their lifejackets. Being new, I tied the leg straps, [which] later saved me. [The] rest of the crew did not [do] this, as it hindered movement. All of the jackets found later had all straps tied, except the leg straps, [which caused the] kapoc [to be] blown out."[15]

By the time Culp and his 52-footer arrived, the weather conditions had worsened: "Cloud cover thickened and lowered. As the seas rose, intermittent severe rain with extreme wind gusts created a very uncomfortable situation." Murray recalled that while the U.S. Coast Guard crew discussed how to pass the towline to the fishing vessel, the line to *Mermaid* slackened. The crew of *Mermaid* took this as the signal to throw off the towline to the 40-footer. There were now four vessels in confused seas and 250 feet of towline floating around "looking for a nice shaft to wrap around," Murray recalled. "Terry immediately commenced pulling [in] the line, Acie grabbed Terry['s] belt and a stanchion and held on." Murray slowly maneuvered the 40-footer clear of the line.

Meanwhile, Culp's crew managed to get another line to *Mermaid*. While all this was taking place, all the craft "were being [shoved] rapidly" to the northwest, and the surf of Peacock Spit "was extremely close."[16]

Swells were now breaking across the channel and the wind was blowing a steady thirty-five to forty knots from the south-southwest. Communications between the boats at the scene became even more difficult. The radios on board the Cape Disappointment boats, soaked by the seas, made them almost "worthless."[17] Culp contacted Senior Chief Berto and discussed the situation. Berto later recalled the impression that Culp intended to tow *Mermaid* to the Columbia River Lightship, located approximately seven miles off the south jetty, and await better bar conditions. Culp instead changed his mind and decided to cross the bar. The three U.S. Coast Guard boats set out for the bar, with *Mermaid* under tow by *Triumph*.

Murray in the 40-footer led the way. Originally, his plan called for him to ease slowly up to the bar, evaluate the conditions and then decide where to cross. The seas now made crossing Murray's only option. Edwards, in the 36-footer, followed at "several hundred yards" on Murray's right quarter. Seaman Edwards planned to cover Murray and provide any necessary help. Culp, at the wheel of *Triumph* and towing *Mermaid*, followed several hundred yards from Murray's port quarter.

On board the 40-footer, Murray's crewman, Lowe, tried to repair the radio in the cabin, which, in the close confines, required that he take off his bulky lifejacket. Outside the cabin, on the coxswain flat near Murray, Maxwell hung on. Maxwell wore a lifejacket, Murray did not. This may seem incredible to modern readers, but the bulky Navy-style lifejacket of the day, combined with the foul weather gear of 1961, made a coxswain's work almost impossible in rough bar crossings. "Under rough bar conditions," the official investigation explained, "it is necessary for the coxswains of these boats to keep working the throttle, to steady the wheel by putting body pressure on it, to occasionally use the spotlights and radios and at the same time to hang on to maintain balance. They find it difficult to do all this with a bulky lifejacket fully rigged over heavy foul weather gear." Murray kept his lifejacket nearby, ready for quick donning. He peered through the low visibility and high seas. Later, at the official hearing on the rescue, the boatswain's mate related that he thought he could make a safe crossing.

By now, the three U.S. Coast Guard boats had lost sight of one another. Murray pushed the throttle forward and started across the bar. At buoy number 7, a series of three "extremely large swells" approached the 40-footer from the stern. Murray successfully maneuvered his boat through the first two swells, but the third broke just as it reached the stern of the boat. The wave picked up the stern, and the boat surfed down the swell at a high rate of speed. Murray grabbed his lifejacket and slipped it on. The bow of the 40-footer plowed into the sea, throwing its stern high into the air and catapulting the boat end over end.

The boat launched Maxwell into the water. Surfacing, he spotted the overturned 40-footer, swam to the capsized craft, crawled up onto the stern, and clung to the propeller shaft. Lowe found himself upside down in a flooding cabin. At first disoriented, he worked his way to the hatch and escaped, surfacing some ten feet from the boat. He swam to the utility boat and joined Maxwell on the stern.

Murray, at the wheel, found himself underwater beneath the boat, his lifejacket's leg straps caught on the coxswain's flat. He could not free himself; he felt completely "helpless and [with a] complete lack of control." It seemed like "a lifetime," he later recalled, "but was not a second" until he grabbed his knife and cut the strap. He felt "overwhelming joy" when his hand broke the surface of the water some thirty or forty feet astern of the overturned boat. Murray had swallowed a great deal of water and had become "exhausted." The balsa life raft from the 40-footer broke free and drifted near him. He reached the raft but "couldn't hang onto it." As he explained later, he "wove" his "right arm [through] the webbing." A wave picked up the raft and carried it to the stern of the utility boat. The first sounds Murray heard turned out to be "Acie and Terry calling for help."[18]

Edwards, in the 36-footer, worried about the loss of a visual sighting of the 40-footer. He also was very concerned about his motor lifeboat. Both the engine and rudder were sluggish. Another check of the stern compartment showed it half full of water. On reaching the vicinity of buoy number 7, Edwards decided to make for the lightship. While turning the wheel for the lightship, a crewman on the 36-footer spotted the overturned 40-footer, with its crew clinging to the stern. Edwards maneuvered the 36-footer toward the stern of the 40-footer. Lowe leaped into the water and swam to the motor lifeboat. Edwards backed away and started his second approach. A breaker caught the 36-footer and slammed it into the overturned boat. The motor lifeboat crew pulled their two shipmates on board. Once Murray and his crew were safely on board, Edwards radioed a Mayday call, the international radio call of distress. Knowing his radio was weak, he asked anyone within hearing to notify the Cape Disappointment Station that the 40-footer had capsized and the U.S. Coast Guardsmen were on board the 36-footer. Edwards informed the station he was making for the lightship. Senior Chief Berto received the call and immediately ordered his two 36-footers to the scene.

Murray took over the wheel of the 36-footer. He first thought about salvaging the 40-footer, but the collision had caused additional flooding on board the motor lifeboat. It would be only a matter of time before the water reached the engine. Abandoning any thoughts of salvaging, Murray shaped a course to the lightship. Exhausted, Murray turned the wheel back to Edwards. Shortly after that, everyone on board the 36-footer momentarily spotted the 52-footer inbound with *Mermaid* in tow.

Suddenly, a large breaker approached the 36-foot motor lifeboat. Edwards backed down to meet it, but the engine faltered. Edwards now had to keep the engine at full throttle to keep it from quitting. This caused the lifeboat to take a beating from the waves. After a "harrowing" trip of over an hour, the 36-footer arrived at the lightship with its stern awash, its engine compartment almost half full of water, and its rudder control "practically gone." The only dry compartment was the forward one. Nevertheless, the 36-foot motor lifeboat had brought its six U.S. Coast Guardsmen to safety. The six scrambled on board the lightship, leaving their motor lifeboat moored to the light vessel's stern. The heavy seas made it impossible to pump out the boat, and within twenty minutes only its bow was visible. It sank at the mooring line at 5:45 A.M., and "the mooring line subsequently went slack."

Culp, on board the 52-foot motor lifeboat, started to experience trouble. Shortly after he took over the tow near buoy 1, the towline parted. Culp maneuvered the 52-footer back to *Mermaid.* Over the radio, he discussed rigging a bridle, a towing arrangement to make a tow track behind the towing vessel. By this time the *Mermaid* was drifting too far to the left side of the channel and dangerously close to Peacock Spit. This ruled out the extra time needed to rig a bridle.[19] Culp's crew again passed and secured the four-inch manila towing hawser to *Mermaid.* To prevent the line from chaffing on the forward rail of the fishing vessel, *Mermaid*'s crew slipped "a rubber tire" beneath the line. Culp again began his tow along the "black buoy line," the inbound left side of the channel. It was at this time that Murray on board the 36-footer had glimpsed *Triumph* and its tow. A few minutes later, the towline again parted at *Mermaid*'s bow. Shortly after 8:00 P.M., Culp radioed that the towline had parted, that *Mermaid* was drifting into the breakers in Peacock Spit, and that he was "going in to get him." At 8:13, the U.S. Coast Guard stations on the Columbia River received an emergency radio call from *Mermaid.* The owner of the boat, Bert E. Bergman, reported that *Triumph* had capsized. Only one of the motor lifeboat's crew had managed to reach the fishing vessel. Again *Mermaid* was drifting toward Peacock Spit and Bergman said they needed help "urgently."

Senior Chief Berto at Point Adams called the district about the situation. The district RCC dispatched the cutter *Yocona* (WAT-168), moored at Astoria, and the cutter *Modoc* (WMEC-194), at Coos Bay, Oregon, to get underway to the scene.

Chief Porter, at Cape Disappointment, managed to raise *Mermaid* by radio and speak with *Triumph* crewman, Petrin. In a state of shock, Engineman Petrin reported, "Chief, a big breaker hit us and the 52-footer went down. I am the only one left." At just about this time, the Columbia River pilot boat *Peacock,* a 138-foot vessel with James C. Messer, the mate, on watch, was outbound in the channel at buoy number 4, about one and a half miles from the scene. Messer heard *Mermaid*'s distress call. He saw the fishing vessel in "extremely" rough water near buoy number 5. Bergman, on board *Mermaid,* saw *Peacock* and called "several times" asking the vessel to come over and pass them a line. Messer debated the wisdom of taking his vessel into such waters. Five to ten minutes later, while still undecided, someone on board the 36-footer contacted Messer, informing him they were making for the lightship in a damaged condition, with six people on board. Messer felt it more important to "concern himself with the safety of six men on the 36-foot lifeboat than the three men on the [*Mermaid*]." He then joined the 36-footer and escorted it to the lightship.

On board *Triumph* when the motor lifeboat capsized, Engineman Gordon E. Huggins was below decks in the after compartment. When the 52-footer took over the tow of *Mermaid,* Huggins developed a "terrific nosebleed" and went below.[20] Gordon F. Sussex was also in the forward compartment. Huggins left the compartment to go into the aft compartment when Sussex became seasick. Huggins heard the towline being put out. Shortly afterward, Petrin opened the hatch leading to the aft compartment and yelled to Huggins to get a heaving line. Soon after bringing the line to Petrin, Huggins heard the towline go out again. A little later, he felt the motor lifeboat make an unusually sharp roll to starboard. He was not frightened because his shipmates had told him the boat would always right itself.[21]

But the roll did not stop. Huggins found himself sitting on the compartment's overhead, with deck planking and gear from the boatswain's locker falling all around him. He went to the companionway and tried to open the watertight door. Blocked. Huggins noticed water coming into the compartment. He went back to the lazaret. The engines of *Triumph* continued for a few minutes, then died. The compartment's lighting went out. Fumbling in the dark, the engineman searched and found a portable battery-operated lantern and the fire axe stowed near the compartment's hatch. He tied a lifejacket to the lantern so he would not lose it, then swung the axe, hoping to chop his way out. Disoriented, Huggins only managed to chop some side paneling of the compartment. The lifeboat rocked slowly for ten to twenty minutes.

Huggins now faced the nightmare of all sailors: a flooding compartment and no way out. But as the water rose, the boat rolled again, this time righting itself. Water drained away from Huggins into the bilge. He made his way out onto the main deck. The motor lifeboat rode normally, but down by its head. Huggins tried to open the hatch into the forward compartment but found it jammed. He decided to try to start the engine. He opened the hatch to the engine room and started down the ladder, but half way down he heard water sloshing below him. That amount of water, he knew, would make it impossible to restart the engines, and even if he could restart them, he might again find himself trapped below decks. He did not know how to anchor the motor lifeboat and he could not find any flares. He made his way back up the stairs and determined that his only course of action was to go to the lee of the after companionway and wait. The seas worsened and *Triumph* continued to go down by the head. An hour later, the motor lifeboat took another steep roll and disappeared after throwing Huggins into the water. He had his lifejacket on and felt himself thrown about "violently in breaking seas." Huggins saw a nearby aircraft drop flares. "I knew they couldn't get to me," he later recalled. "I thought it was the end."[22] Shortly after that, he felt the bottom of Peacock Spit. Spotting lights, Huggins began calling for help.

Back at the Cape Disappointment Station, Chief Porter, upon hearing about the capsizing, began organizing beach patrols. In short order, Porter received calls from the Ilwaco Fire Department, the local Washington State Highway Patrol, and the local state fisheries commission, all offering volunteers to help search the beaches. At 10:45 P.M., one group of searchers found Huggins near the beach, three-quarters of a mile north of the north jetty. Thirty years after the incident, Huggins remembered that Junior Myer and Grover Dillard from the North Head Light Station pulled him out of the water. "We heard him screaming for help," Myer remembered. "I ran to the surf. He was getting thrashed about." Myer grabbed Huggins and pulled him over logs strewn upon the beach. "I don't remember being scared," Myer said. "You just do what you have to do."[23] After that, rescuers transported Huggins to the Ilwaco hospital. At 12:15 A.M., searchers also found the body of Boatswain's Mate John L. Culp close to where Huggins had washed ashore.

The two 36-footer motor lifeboats from Point Adams arrived on scene. One of the motor lifeboats diverted to the Cape Disappointment Station to pick up Boatswain's Mate 1st Class John C. Webb, the officer in charge of the North Head Light Station. Webb had six years of experience at the Point Adams Station, and Senior Chief Berto considered him "the most experienced lifeboat coxswain in the Columbia River area." Webb had called Berto and volunteered to help. Senior Chief Berto authorized Webb to relieve Boatswain's Mate 1st Class Hernando Lopez as coxswain of the CG-36554.

At 9:10 P.M., at least an hour after the capsizing of *Triumph*, the crew of the CG-36535 located *Mermaid* drifting near buoy 7. Interestingly, Boatswain's Mate 1st Class Willis P. Miller, who should have been on board *Triumph*, was now coxswain of the third boat towing *Mermaid*. Miller and his crew worked the fishing vessel from the location of the capsizing to near the buoy. The crew of the CG-36535 passed a three-and-a-half-inch manila towline to *Mermaid*. Miller shaped a course toward the lightship. Strong winds, heavy seas, and a flood tide proved too much for the 36-footer. The elements shoved both craft almost due east across the channel. On board *Mermaid*, the crew secured the manila hawser through its starboard bow chock. The fishing vessel kept veering sharply to port, making it "very difficult to keep up into the wind and sea." At 9:45 P.M., the two craft crossed over "an exceptionally large swell which was just on the verge of breaking." The swell's full force caught *Mermaid.* The towline on board the motor lifeboat "surged violently on the towing bitts, then snapped with a jolt that threw the entire crew of the CG-36535 to the deck. When they looked back . . . [*Mermaid*] had disappeared."

At just this time, Capt. Kenneth H. McAlpin was piloting the SS *Diaz de Solis* outbound near buoy 8. The Pilots Association had earlier called and told McAlpin to anchor inside because of bar conditions. McAlpin, however, felt it safer to continue outbound. At three hundred yards off *Mermaid,* the pilot could see the towing operation. He watched as the 36-footer crossed a large swell with *Mermaid* in tow. Immediately afterward, the swell broke over *Mermaid* and the vessel "seemed to be thrown end over end." It disappeared. Captain McAlpin used the ship's searchlights to illuminate the area and maneuvered *Diaz de Solis* to create a lee for the searching CG-36535. After fifteen minutes, the searchlights burned out. Captain McAlpin felt it too dangerous to remain in the vicinity and ordered *Diaz de Solis* across the bar.

At 8:57 P.M., forty-one minutes after receiving the call from the Rescue Coordination Center, the cutter *Yocona* got underway from Astoria. The cutter was near buoy 19 when it received Miller's call that *Mermaid* had capsized. *Yocona* arrived near buoy 8 at the time CG-36554 joined the other 36-footer in searching the area. The cutter began illuminating the area with its searchlight. A U.S. Coast Guard fixed-wing aircraft on a training flight from San Francisco to U.S. Coast Guard Air Station Port Angeles, Washington, diverted and began dropping flares. Later, other fixed-wing aircraft from Port Angeles also dropped illumination flares. At 2:30 A.M., the two 36-footers returned to Point Adams, while the cutter *Yocona* continued the search until daylight.

Beach searches continued. The body of Bert E. Bergman, owner of *Mermaid,* was found on the beach eighteen miles north of the north jetty on 19 January. Petrin's body was the only one not recovered over the days following the incident. The searches ended on 26 January.

Since 1876, the largest loss experienced by one station was seven crewmen. The loss of the five U.S. Coast Guardsmen on board *Triumph* is one of four times, since that year, that the U.S. Coast Guard has lost this many people.[24] The official investigation into the *Mermaid* case exonerated all U.S. Coast Guard personnel. Three officers made up the investigation, headed by captain, and future commandant of the U.S. Coast Guard, Williard J. Smith. The officers seemed willing to side with the men who were in the boats that terrible night.[25]

There are at least two memorials to the *Mermaid* case in the Ilwaco area, one in a nearby park and the other at the nearby Cape Disappointment Station. A plaque dedicated to the crew of *Triumph* hangs on the mess deck of the Cape Disappointment Station. Another plaque hangs on the wall outside the commanding officer's office. The *Mermaid* case also is part of an exhibit at the Columbia River Maritime Museum at Astoria, in a display that features the U.S. Coast Guard on the river.

John C. Culp posthumously received the Gold Life Saving Medal. Members of Culp's crew who perished, John Hoban, Joseph E. Petrin, Ralph E. Mace, and Gordon F. Sussex, posthumously received the Silver Life Saving Medal. The only survivor of the *Triumph*, Gordon E. Huggins, also received the Silver Life Saving Medal.

Larry B. Edwards, coxswain of the 36-footer who rescued the 40-footer crew, received the Gold Life Saving Medal. Darrell J. Murray, Willis P. Miller, and John C. Webb received the Coast Guard Commendation Medal (Webb's second such medal for valor). The other crewmen on board the 40-footer and 36-footers received commandant's letters of commendation.[26]

In 1982, twenty-one years after the incident, Senior Chief Darrell Murray, U.S. Coast Guard (Ret.), coxswain of the 40-footer, wrote to U.S. Coast Guard headquarters for a transcript of the investigation into the *Mermaid* case for a claim to the Veteran's Administration but failed to receive a response. He then wrote to his U.S. senator. The response from headquarters to the senator said, "We have conducted a thorough search of our files of such investigations, both at U.S. Coast Guard Headquarters and the Thirteenth Coast Guard District Office in Seattle, Washington. Although every possible subject category was searched, we have, unfortunately, been unable to find any record related to the incident to which Mr. Murray referred." In other words, the case did not exist. In only twenty-one years, the leadership of the U.S. Coast Guard had allowed a major loss within their service to slip from their institutional memory. Senior Chief Murray on his own managed to locate a copy of the investigation within a unit located in the Thirteenth District. Murray had the document reproduced and, along with photocopied newspaper clippings related to the case, distributed to some U.S. Coast Guard locations. Incredibly, in a 1990 request concerning the *Mermaid* case, the U.S. Coast Guard's Thirteenth District again reported having no record of the case.[27]

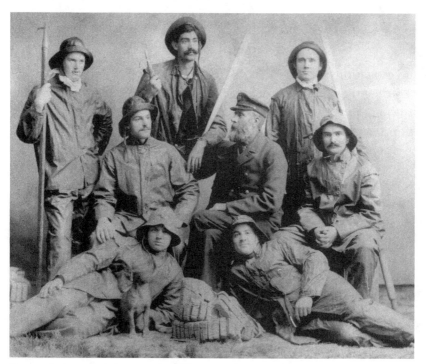

Keeper Lawrence O. Lawson (*middle, second row*) and his crew of student lifesavers at the U.S. Life-Saving Service station at Evanston, Illinois. In his later years, Lawson sported a much longer beard.

U.S. Coast Guard

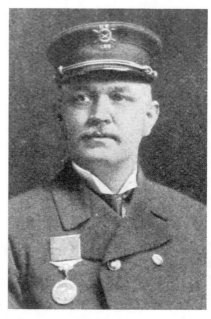

Keeper W. W. Griesser of the U.S. Life-Saving Service Station at Buffalo, New York, received the Gold Life Saving Medal for his swimming battle of three-quarters of an hour to rescue a man from the frigid waters of Lake Erie in November 1900.

U.S. Coast Guard

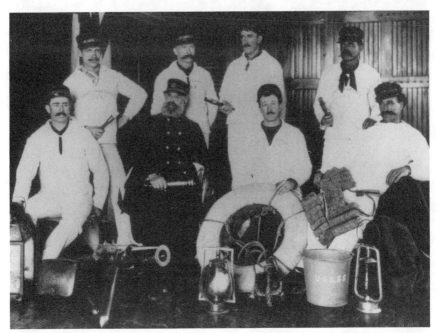

Keeper Joshua James (*seated, second from left*), the most famous lifesaver in the U.S. Life-Saving Service era.

U.S. Coast Guard

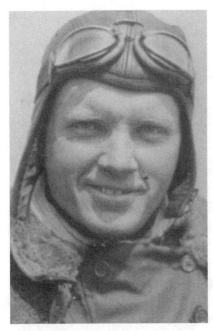

Cdr. C. C. Von Paulson, an early pilot in the U.S. Coast Guard and one of the few pilots to earn the Gold Life Saving Medal.

U.S. Coast Guard

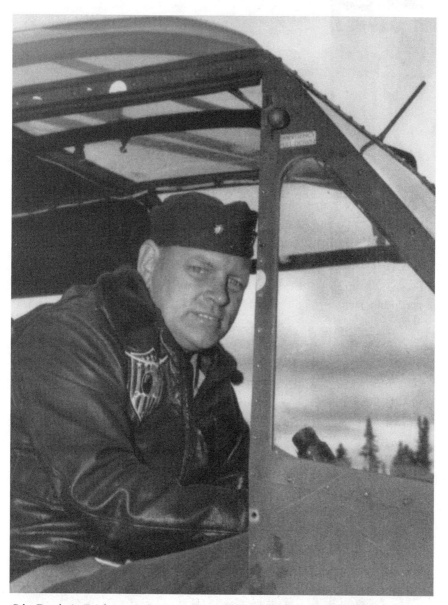

Cdr. Frank A. Erickson at the controls of an HNS-1 helicopter in 1947.
U.S. Coast Guard

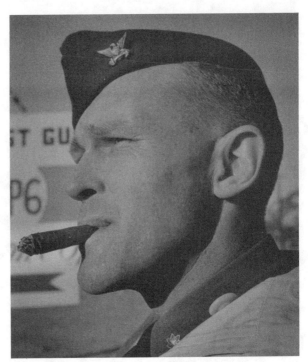

Cdr. Donald B. MacDiarmid, an expert in the use of seaplanes for search and rescue in the U.S. Coast Guard.

U.S. Coast Guard

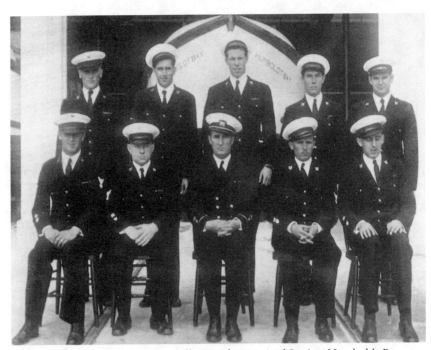

Warrant Officer Garner J. Churchill (*seated, center*) of Station Humboldt Bay, California.

U.S. Coast Guard

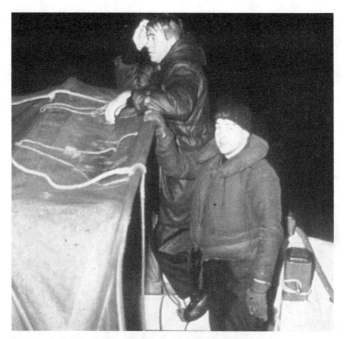

Boatswain's Mate 1st Class Bernard C. Webber, without a cap, and Seaman Erving E. Maske after the amazing rescue of sailors from *Pendelton*.

Photograph by Richard C. Kelsey, Chatham, Massachusetts; courtesy Cape Cod Community College

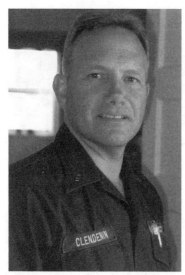

Chief Warrant Officer F. Scott Clendenin while commanding officer of the Yaquina Bay Station, Oregon.

Courtesy of F. Scott Clendenin

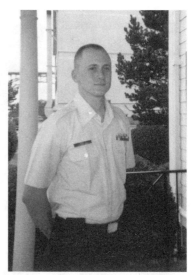

Boatswain's Mate 3d Class Michael Carola received the Coast Guard Medal for his work on the case of *Little Fly Fisherman* near Station Oregon Inlet, North Carolina, in 2000.

Courtesy of Dennis L. Noble

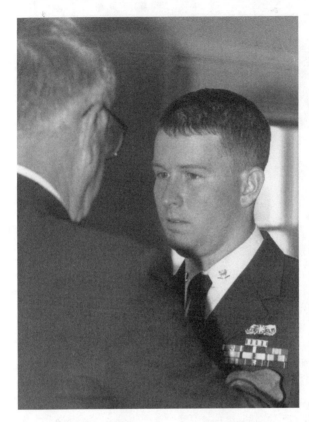

Boatswain's Mate 3d Class Michael L. Dunning receives the Coast Guard Medal for his rescue of a woman from the pleasure boat *Doormat*, near Montauk, New York, in 1993.

U.S. Coast Guard

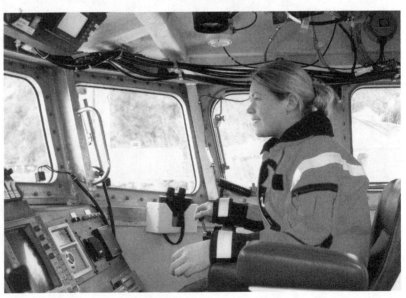

Boatswain's Mate 2d Class Beth Rassmussen at the inside steering station of a 47-foot motor lifeboat at Station Cape Disappointment, Washington.

Courtesy of AST2 Allen Aurichio, U.S. Coast Guard

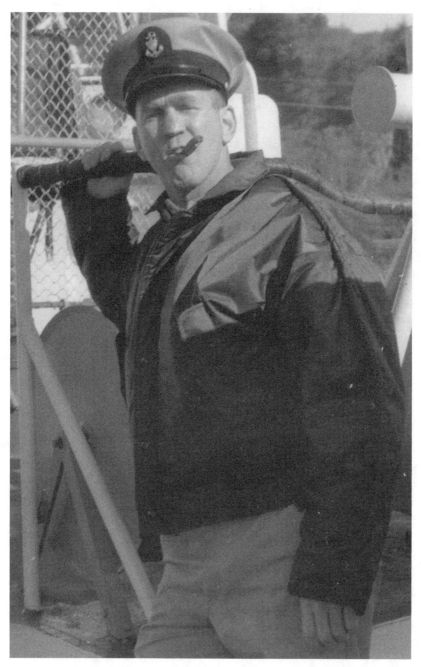

Master Chief Boatswain's Mate Thomas D. McAdams, U.S. Coast Guard (Ret.), earlier in his career. McAdams, a legend in the service, is shown aboard a 44-foot motor lifeboat and with his ever-present cigar.

U.S. Coast Guard

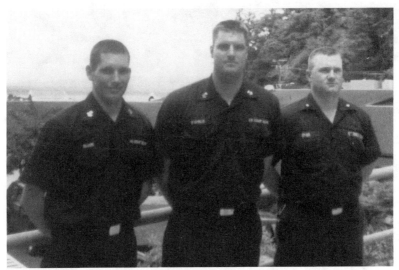

Left to right: Boatswain's Mate 2d Class Scott E. Slade, Boatswain's Mate 1st Class Christopher D'Amelio, and Machinery Technician 3d Class Darrell M. Ryan of Station Cape Disappointment, Washington.

Courtesy of Dennis L. Noble

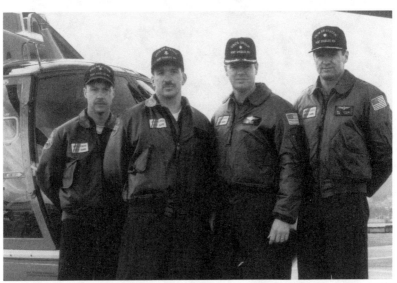

Aircrew of helicopter 6589 (*left to right*): Neal Amos, Charles S. Carter, Raymond J. Miller, and Paul Langlois. Amos, Miller, and Langlois received the Distinguished Flying Cross for their work; Carter received the U.S. Coast Guard Commendation Medal.

U.S. Coast Guard

PART III
1965–1995

10 | It Is a Rewarding Job

In 1961, the same year of the *Mermaid* rescue, the U.S. Coast Guard began to develop a new heavy weather motor lifeboat. The 44-footer, made of Corten steel, had twin propellers powered by twin diesel engines, making it an easier boat to handle than the old 36-footer. In the new motor lifeboat, the coxswain sat amidship in a chair and a strong windshield protected the crew. This does not mean, however, that crews would not get wet during heavy weather. Far from it. But unlike its predecessors, the boat provided the crew some protection from the sea. When new, the boat could make fifteen knots, but after years of use, the typical cruising speed was only twelve knots.

Like the old 36-footer, the boat was at first viewed skeptically by many old lifeboatmen, but it eventually became accepted and loved by those at the stations. Like its predecessors, the 44-footer was self-righting and self-bailing. Crewmembers (four per boat) could strap themselves into safety belts, called surfbelts, and then snap the belts into D rings placed throughout the boat.[1]

From 1964 to 1995, the U.S. Coast Guard also developed other boats for the rescue stations. The 41-footer, with a crew of three, was designed for inshore and some offshore work in moderate seas. With an aluminum hull and twin diesels, its cruising speed was eighteen knots and its top speed twenty-one knots. Also at stations with heavy surf, the service had a 30-foot surf rescue boat (SRB) for two-man crews. SRBs dashed into the surf, their crews grabbed survivors, and they dashed back out again. The SRB had a single screw and a top speed of thirty-one knots. In the late 1990s, the service started phasing out this boat.[2]

THERE'S A BABY IN THE WATER

On Monday, 21 November 1977, the morning watch at the U.S. Coast Guard station at Ashtabula, Ohio, faced a cold, drizzly day. At 9:36 A.M., a police officer telephoned the communications watchstander with the news that someone had just thrown a baby into the frigid waters of the Ashtabula River. The watchstander immediately pressed the SAR alarm, beginning a twenty-minute rescue that would involve nine men and an eleven-month-old baby.

Boatswain's Mate 1st Class John P. Johnson, twenty-nine, with eight years in the U.S. Coast Guard, started a crew toward the 44-foot motor lifeboat. At just this time, Chief Boatswain's Mate Robert G. Edwards, thirty-eight, a nineteen-year veteran and the officer in charge, arrived to take over.

"There was the normal amount of confusion," Chief Edwards later related. "I told the boat crew to get going and Johnson to take at least two men with him, take the pickup and head out to the end of the [coal loading] dock. I then questioned the watchstander on what information he had received over the telephone and then passed the additional information by radio to the boat."[3]

Boatswain's Mate 3d Class Richard Alexander, twenty-four, had just started his cleaning detail when the SAR alarm echoed off the station's walls. He sprinted toward the motor lifeboat. Once aboard, he switched on the radio and tuned it to channel 21. The radio brought the news of a baby in the water.

Seaman Apprentice (Boatswain's Mate) Keith A. Roberts, eighteen, with only six months in the U.S. Coast Guard, was doing what sailors have done for years: swabbing the deck. On hearing the alarm, he ran down the stairs and started toward the boat. "I saw our coxswain running, so I said to myself, 'If he's running, I'd better be ready,'" he recalled.

Fireman William R. Cooper, twenty, heard the alarm and ran down the hall. He saw Chief Edwards waving everybody out. "There's a baby in the water! Go!" yelled the chief.

"I was boat engineer that day," recalled Cooper, "and was the first one in the boat and got the engines started and when Alex, the boat coxswain, was on the boat we were able to fire off right away."

Seaman Joel Hibel, twenty, although off duty, jumped onto the boat and joined Alexander, Cooper, and Roberts as the boat left the station. Meanwhile, Johnson told two crewmen, Randy Phillips and Mark Clark, to come with him in the station's pickup truck. "I took the truck and two fellows and headed for the scene," recalled Johnson. "We did not know at this time if it was an infant in the water, or a doll, or a false alarm, but we activated every bit of resources we had."

An eighth of a mile from the station, Johnson dropped off Phillips and Clark "at the end of a line of railroad cars, and they ran down the dock checking the shoreline." Johnson "continued down the dock with the truck for another quarter of a mile."

Alexander, the motor lifeboat coxswain, recalled that as he headed toward the pier, the river "had maybe a half a foot of waves in it, rippling pretty good and the weather was chilly. The first thing that I saw [when near the scene] was the men on the shore pointing over toward an area we had just passed. I began to turn the boat around."

Alexander handled the boat. Roberts, with the help of Hibel, donned the wet suit then used by crewmen to protect themselves from exposure should they have to enter the cold water. Both Hibel and Roberts then made their way to the bow of the motor lifeboat.

"We saw our people on the shore pointing and yelling, 'Right here! Right here!'" said Roberts. "They were telling us to turn around, turn around. As we made the turn, one of our engines stalled . . . and it made it kind of hard to maneuver, but by the time we got to the end of the turn, Cooper had the engine running. We crept up to where the baby was. Joel Hibel thought it was a doll."

Hibel said, "I saw something floating. I pointed at it and said to Alex, "'That's it!'"

"I corrected the engine," recalled Cooper, "and Alexander turned around and we saw [the two crewmen] on the wall waving us over there. I went to the bow with Roberts. We didn't know whether it was a doll or a baby. Roberts took one look, said it was a baby and jumped in."

The eighteen-year-old Roberts recalled, "I remember that it shocked me when I saw the baby, but I didn't let that stop me. I just jumped off. It was just a reaction from seeing the baby. I don't remember feeling the thirty-nine-degree water, but I do remember praying while I was swimming toward the baby.

"Alexander put the boat about two feet in front of us so that the boat blocked off the wind and that helped a lot. I grabbed the baby and swam toward the shore. I tried to get ahold of the seawall, but it was kind of slimy and too high for me to grab. So I grabbed Mark Clark's hand and then passed the baby with my other hand to where Cooper could grab the baby. Randy Phillips then grabbed my hand and both pulled me up, they're pretty big guys.

"William Cooper took the baby and laid it on something and started to give mouth-to-mouth resuscitation."

"When Roberts went into the water," Cooper later recalled, "for a few seconds I sort of lost myself and got pretty upset, but then I sort of pulled my stuff together and leaped to the wall when Alexander got the boat alongside the wall.

"When the two guys on the wall grabbed Roberts, I took the baby from them and looked around for a split second and all that I saw that was handy and flat was a railroad tie. I laid the baby on the tie longways and she just limped over it and it scared me even more. That's when I proceeded to clear her throat and started mouth-to-mouth.

"I think I was crying and the only thing going through my mind was to save the baby. I didn't think whether she was dead or not. I guess I took it for granted that there was life in her. I just wanted to revive her. . . . That's all I could think about. While I was giving mouth-to-mouth, John Johnson arrived."

"As I came down the dock," Johnson recalled, "an Ashtabula police car was racing alongside of me. I saw the 44-foot boat was already there and the guys were bent over the dock on their bellies. Roberts was passing the infant to Cooper, who laid it across a railroad tie. . . The infant just drooped like it was a limp noodle. It just fell there.

"The baby was dark purple in color, except for its fatty parts of the thighs and stomach, but the lips, ears, fingers and toes were a deep purple. We were a good ways off the main road and I immediately made the decision that we needed to get the baby to a hospital without waiting for an ambulance, I did not know how long it would be before an ambulance or something got there. I decided to use the police car.

"I then picked up the baby, with Cooper still giving mouth-to-mouth, and headed for the car. We climbed over a bunch of rocks to get to it and entered the cruiser. Once we got into the car and started down the dock, I felt the throat and groin and under the armpits for a heartbeat. Not finding any, I gave the baby a good jolt and started CPR. We were holding the infant about chest high in order to make it easy to tilt the head back and give mouth-to-mouth. I gave CPR and Cooper gave mouth-to-mouth.

"The [policeman] proceeded down the dock and streets at a high rate of speed. I remember him yelling and cussing at the people who weren't listening to the siren and not moving out of the way. Other than that, Cooper and I tried to place our interest on proper procedures to save the infant."

"I can't even remember the place where the baby had been thrown into the water, don't even remember where we were," Cooper recounted. "I only remember it was quite rough giving mouth-to-mouth to the baby while going through the coal dock area, the car bounced so much I had a hard time keeping my mouth on hers. I remember seeing how her eyes were dilated and in the background I could sort of hear the policeman cussin' at the drivers, yelling at them to get out of the way."

"We arrived at the hospital," Johnson remembered. "I did not even stop to open the door, the [policeman] came around and opened [it] for us and we ran right into the emergency room. One of the doctors from the cold water drown team took over the CPR, but Cooper kept up the mouth-to-mouth for another thirty to forty-five seconds before he was relieved by a doctor with a respirator. Up to this time, Cooper and myself didn't have time to let our feelings enter into what we were doing. After being relieved, it wasn't until four or five minutes [later] that the doctor said, 'We have a real good, strong heartbeat.'"

"I was pretty upset in the hospital," recalled Cooper, "and was pacing the floor. All the time we were waiting I was afraid she was going to die. I don't know what I would have done. I'd have felt that I hadn't performed my job. I remember when they got the heartbeat detector. They put it on her and the nurse came up to us and pointed out the heartbeat. I heard the beat on the beeper and that was pretty exciting."

"The doctor said, 'It looks like she's going to make it,'" recalled Johnson. "And at that time Willie and I hugged each other and, you know, we burst into tears with happiness."

The next morning, eleven-month-old Cassy Marie was up and playing. Later, the crew of the Ashtabula Station repeated what many who work in maritime rescue say: "The happiness of saving a life is rewarding enough, it is a rewarding job when you can do something like this."

INTO THE INFERNO

Five members of the U.S. Coast Guard station at Southwest Harbor, Maine, boarded their 41-foot utility boat, CG-41439, for an assignment on the night of 31 August 1991. The five drew the duty of providing a safety zone around a barge used as a platform for a fireworks display at Northeast Harbor. Sometimes fate seems to help lifesavers. The CG-41439's fire monitor, the device used to spray water on a fire, needed repair, so Southwest Harbor Station borrowed another one from Rockland Station. The coxswain of the boat, Boatswain's Mate 2d Class Paul J. Dupuis, "just to be safe," mounted the borrowed monitor and tested it. Instead of stowing it, Dupuis decided to leave it mounted. Years later, Dupuis recalled that this "was the [first] time I've ever had a monitor mounted while doing a security zone."[4]

The night's duty started as planned. Fireworks lit the dark sky, and the harbor echoed with loud claps and voices of exclamation at the display. Suddenly, sparks from the display ignited a stock of pyrotechnics on the deck of the barge, and a huge fireball erupted. Three people aboard the barge leaped into the water.[5]

Dupuis quickly maneuvered the 41-footer close to the barge. Because the water monitor was in place, Dupuis recalled, his crew "literally was pumping water . . . within 30 seconds of the [first] explosion." Boat engineer Machinery Technician 3d Class Bruce E. Sherwood started the boat's fire pump then grabbed a heaving line to throw to the men in the water.

Dupuis recalled the main "problem we had . . . was we didn't know how many people were on the barge . . . and as we pulled people from the water my crew was asking them how many people [were on the barge]. In their dazed state, they didn't know.

"When we [first] pulled up to the barge, we did not know that people were still on it. There [were too] many fireworks and fires around to be able to see them. After my reservist, [Port Securityman 3d Class] Brian Baker, put some water on the barge, I finally saw [a] man on deck [through] the flames. . . . I was behind the relative safety of the windshield and was able to look around better than those on deck dodging fireworks. The only thing I yelled was, 'There's a guy right there!' The 41[-footer] was about 3 or 4 feet from the barge so I engaged the engine and put the bow up against it, Bruce Sherwood and [Seaman Apprentice] Carol [A.] James took it from there."[6]

The U.S. Coast Guard crew knew that secondary explosions were inevitable. Despite the danger, Sherwood, also an emergency medical technician (EMT), grabbed his EMT kit and leaped aboard the barge. Somehow he managed to get the injured man to his feet and aboard the CG-41439. Once aboard, Sherwood started first aid on the man.

At almost the same time as Sherwood leaped aboard the barge, James threw a life ring overboard to a man in the water then grabbed another line and threw it to yet another man in the water. After she helped pull both men into the boat, she helped another crewman move the stokes litter (a metal stretcher with sides) and other medical equipment from the lower cabin to the main deck. Without thinking of her own safety, James then jumped to the barge to help her shipmates move the victims.

Another crewman, Seaman Robert A. Bowen, manned the fire monitor at the 41-footer's bow. As Dupuis maneuvered the boat closer to the inferno, Bowen applied water to the burning man and the deck fire. Once he knocked down the flames, Bowen helped James with the medical equipment from the lower cabin. Then he, too, disregarding his own safety, jumped aboard the barge.

The other member of the boat crew, Baker, a reservist on active duty, grabbed a heaving line and threw it to another person in the water. Baker then pulled a victim aboard the boat. Showing the same courage as his shipmates, Baker leaped aboard the barge and helped victims to the boat. He next went back to the fire monitor to put more water on the fire.

Dupuis recalled that once all the survivors and his crew were aboard, "I was starting to back away as Baker continue to apply water to the barge. I heard him yell a couple of superlatives followed by a 'get out of here!' At about the same time, it went up."[7]

Viewing a photograph of the large mushroom-shaped fireball on the barge, one wonders how anyone aboard the 41-footer survived. Burning debris and shrapnel flew in all directions. Sherwood used his own body to shelter his patients on the deck of the 41-footer. Baker, at the monitor on the bow, took the full force of the explosion and was hurled backward into the boat's superstructure. He received burns and wounds on his face and legs and a cut on his hand, along with numerous bruises on his body. He rolled off the superstructure to the deck. James rushed to Baker, sheltering him from "burning debris," then helped him back to the well deck with the other patients.

The second explosion disabled the 41-footer's radar and cabin lights, dislodged the radio and clock from their mounts, and filled the cabin interior with smoke. Dupuis recalled that after the second explosion, he "lost some time" and "the next thing I [knew] I was picking myself off the deck and there was paper all over the place [from the fireworks]. After we pulled a little further away, I stopped to check on everyone. Baker had a hole in his calf that was about the size of golf ball. There was a lobster boat that pulled up to us and asked if we needed any help. I asked him to call the group and tell them we need ambulances at Northeast Harbor. We headed in and dropped all the people off.

"Damn Baker still was handling lines with shrapnel in his chest and a hole in his leg. I had to order him to take a ride in the ambulance. That's the only order I had to give the entire night."[8]

Twelve years after the fireworks explosion in Northeast Harbor, Dupuis, now a chief warrant officer, recalled that his crew was "ready to jump on that barge the second that I [could] get them close enough. There was not one word from anyone that didn't have to do with the job at hand."[9]

For their selfless actions, Paul J. Dupuis, Bruce E. Sherwood, Brian P. Baker, Robert A. Bowen, and Carol A. James deservedly received the Coast Guard Medal.

ALL I COULD THINK OF WAS GETTING HIM ON BOARD

On Monday, 22 August 1994, Thomas Palchanes, thirty-seven, owner of the 28-foot sport fishing vessel *Lyl Cyn,* was returning from the Hudson Canyon area with a party of eight on board. About thirty miles off Sandy Hook, New Jersey, a severe storm built up quickly. "It was a very strong storm for this time of year. . . . It came on in a rush," said James Eberwind, a meteorologist for the National Weather Service.[10] As the weather worsened, Palchanes turned for port.

As the seas steadily increased, waves tossed *Lyl Cyn* "about like a toy in a tub," recalled members of the fishing party. Palchanes fought at the wheel to keep his vessel on course. William Reube, one of the fishing party, remembered that "the vessel struggled up swells as high as houses. When it reached the crest of each wave, it would slide down the other side, a dizzying, horrifying plummet that got worse with each mountain of water."

A wave, later estimated at twenty feet, struck *Lyl Cyn* and blew out its windshield. As the craft took on water, the engine quit. Palchanes sent out a radio broadcast for help. Everyone on board the craft donned lifejackets. "We shot off the flares," Reube said. "[The *Lyl Cyn*] went down in a heartbeat. It was done."

A HH-65A Dolphin helicopter from Air Station Brooklyn, New York, spotted the foundering fishing craft thirty miles southeast of Manasquan Inlet, New Jersey. The pilot, Lt. Cdr. David Maxson, battled driving rain and winds steady at thirty-five knots and gusting to forty-five knots. In conditions that Lieutenant Commander Maxson would later describe as "very challenging," the helicopter crew lowered a raft to the people on board the sinking *Lyl Cyn*. The waves made it difficult for the survivors to scramble into the raft. Only three made it into the raft; the others clung to the outside of the raft.

Lt. Anthony R. Gentilella, commanding officer of the 110-foot patrol boat *Bainbridge Island* (WPB-1343), was on patrol off the New Jersey coast when he and his sixteen-man crew received orders to proceed immediately to *Lyl Cyn*'s position. "We increased . . . to our top speed and it took us about an hour to get on scene," recalled Lieutenant Gentilella.

Bainbridge Island arrived just twenty minutes after the helicopter lowered the life raft to the survivors. "There were three in the raft and five hanging on," Gentilella remembered. Seaman James Duffy recalled, "When we came up on scene all we could see was about six feet of the nose of the boat above the water. The lights of the boat were underwater. It was eerie, but when we saw the raft and the people in the water . . . we just forgot about everything else. That's when we went to work and did our thing." This was the first SAR case that Duffy worked on board the cutter. As the crew labored to save the survivors, waves pummeled *Bainbridge Island,* rolling the cutter forty degrees.

Fireman Apprentice Jamison E. Merriam dived into the churning sea and swam at least one hundred feet to the nearest victim. Merriam threw a rescue buoy to the struggling man and then towed him to the raft. The survivor climbed on board the life raft. *Bainbridge Island*'s crew used the line Merriam had passed to the man to tow the raft alongside the patrol boat. Merriam then scrambled on board the cutter.

Three victims made it on board *Bainbridge Island.* One man, David Mark Lawson, "was in desperate need of help." At 270 pounds, he was having trouble climbing up the rope ladder onto the cutter. Lawson's physique and the heavy roll of the patrol boat hampered the crew's efforts to bring the survivor on board. Lawson slipped out of his lifejacket. Seaman Duffy recalled, "I had tunnel vision. I saw [Lawson's] face down in the water and all I could think of was getting him on board."

Lawson began to drift away. Seaman Lawrence R. Beatty dived into the sea, swam at least sixty feet, grabbed the desperate Lawson, and started back to *Bainbridge Island.* Beatty later remembered Lawson telling him he "couldn't breathe and I told him to get some strength. I kept telling him we were friends and we'd rescue him, but he was twice my size." As Seaman Beatty approached the cutter, Lieutenant Gentilella had to back the cutter to avoid "a collision with an oncoming merchant ship, leaving both Beatty and Lawson several hundred feet off the bow." Beatty held Lawson's head above the water and worked his way back toward *Bainbridge Island.* "I tried to keep him close to the boat so we could bring him up, but the boat rolled one way and another."

Duffy dived into the water to help with Lawson. Both Beatty and Duffy tried to get Lawson tied into a stokes litter. The seas and violent rolling of *Bainbridge Island* forced the three men under the cutter. Duffy recalled the harrowing scene: "I'd get the man, get him in the stokes, get him alongside the boat but the swells would take me down. Then the boat would come down on me and I'd lose the man. There was no time between the swells, it was like, bang, bang, bang. It was the most frustrating experience of my life." Both Beatty and Duffy tired. "Eventually," Beatty said, "my crew had to pull me on board because I was very fatigued. They continued trying to rescue him. I passed out." Duffy continued his heroic efforts. Then the cutter passed over them, and when they surfaced, Lawson had drifted away and was lost at sea.

In the meantime, the raft holding the two other victims had drifted away. In the darkness and high seas, Lieutenant Gentilella radioed for another helicopter to help in the search. Located two hours later, the two survivors were found "laying down in the raft. They looked exhausted," said Gentilella.

Much later, Gentilella remarked, "For three hours, it was a battle for us to keep ourselves alive and rescue [the survivors]. It was the worse case I've ever had and will probably be one of the worse we will ever have." The cutter's crew continued to search for Lawson, but soon after daylight broke off and returned to port. "I was so upset I lost the man," Duffy said. "I sat on the floor of the galley, wondering if I had done something wrong or if I could have done more. But we've all come to the conclusion that we did everything we could. We saved seven[,] but that one loss really got to the crew."

Bainbridge Island returned to Sandy Hook, New Jersey, with the survivors of *Lyl Cyn*. Once moored, they met the inevitable attention of television cameras and interviews. Almost as if scripted by a Hollywood writer, as Lieutenant Gentilella and his crew underwent questioning by the media, a U.S. Coast Guard 82-foot patrol boat, *Point Jackson* (WPB-82378), returned from rescuing five survivors from the fishing vessel *Harvey Gamage,* lost in the same storm as *Lyl Cyn*.

For their heroic efforts, Lawrence R. Beatty, James R. Duffy, and Jamison E. Merriam received the Coast Guard Medal. The entire crew of *Bainbridge Island* received the U.S. Coast Guard Unit Commendation, the service's "highest unit level award."[11] When Rear Adm. John Linnon, commander of the U.S. Coast Guard's First District, presented Lieutenant Gentilella with the award, the admiral remarked, "I've gone to sea all of my life, but this was an outstanding, impressive case. When I heard the details, it made the hair stand up on the back of my head."

I WAS JUST THINKING OF SAVING THAT WOMAN'S LIFE

James and Karen Olivieri, from Wallington, New Jersey, were weekend fishing three miles north of Montauk Light, Long Island, New York. On Sunday, 3 October 1993, the fishing season was nearing its end. There was a wave chop of three to four feet. At 3:30 P.M. the wind started to pick up. The Olivieris prepared their 25-foot boat, *Doormat,* for the return to shore.[12]

The couple began pulling in the anchor from the stern of *Doormat.* "I didn't realize the anchor was caught on a lobster troll," said James. "The pressure from the troll lines brought the back of the boat down. Water was breaking in, and then a big-sized wave hit the boat and stalled the engine out. I released the anchor, but it didn't do us any good, the waves just kept hitting us." Karen broadcast two radio calls. She called friends on a nearby boat, *Grumpy,* then the U.S. Coast Guard.

At the U.S. Coast Guard's Montauk Station, the communications watchstander began taking the necessary information from Karen Olivieri when communications ended abruptly. The station dispatched a 41-foot boat, the CG-41342, with Boatswain's Mate 3d Class Michael L. Dunning, from Mount Pleasant, South Carolina, on board. The 82-foot patrol boat *Point Bonita* (WPB-82347), patrolling along the east end of Montauk Point, diverted to the scene to help.

Another wave struck *Doormat* and capsized it, catapulting James into the water. While he struggled to reach the boat, another wave knocked Karen back into the cabin of the overturned boat. "I went down and came right back up in an air pocket," she recalled. James managed to swim to the overturned boat. He made "several" attempts to swim under it but was unsuccessful. He began tapping on the outside of the hull. Ten minutes later, the Olivieris' friends in *Grumpy* arrived and began relaying information to the Montauk Station. The 41-footer arrived ten minutes later.

Upon arrival at the scene, the rescue crew's first thoughts were to get James Olivieri out of the water and into the safety of the 41-footer. James, however, refused to leave the water and continued to bang on the hull of *Doormat*. He yelled to the U.S. Coast Guard crew that his wife was in an air pocket under the boat.

Just about this time, the wind began to rise and the waves increased in height. Petty Officer Colin Redy, the coxswain of the CG-41342, discussed with his crew the options available to them, especially in the face of worsening weather. The nearest diver was at least twenty-five minutes away. Normally, U.S. Coast Guard boat crews learn not to go under an overturned boat, as there is great danger in the boat's sinking and trapping both victim and rescuer. "We all just looked at each other and knew somebody had to go in the water," said Dunning. "I went down below [in the cabin], grabbed the [swim] fins and went in the water." The twenty-two-year-old boatswain's mate was a logical choice: he had three years of U.S. Coast Guard experience and was a recreational diver.

Dunning worked his way along the side of *Doormat*'s hull until he reached the distraught James Olivieri. Dunning's efforts failed to calm Olivieri, who continued pounding on the hull. Dunning could hear Karen inside "screaming and pounding on the inside of the hull." The official report of the incident mentions that Karen, a poor swimmer, was, not surprisingly, "in a state of near panic."

By now, *Point Bonita* had arrived and placed another rescue swimmer into the water to help Dunning. Divers were still at least twenty minutes away. Dunning now had to make a difficult decision. He could hear Karen Olivieri inside yelling about being entangled in line. She said she feared trying to swim out and becoming more entangled. James Olivieri showed signs of developing hypothermia and shock. Karen Olivieri still refused to try to swim out, and her "cries for assistance from inside the hull began to get more frantic." Dunning decided he had to at least check under the boat.

Strands of mooring and fishing line hung from *Doormat*. "My biggest concern going under the boat was getting wrapped up in all the fishing lines," the twenty-two-year-old petty officer said. "I went down twice just to scope out the boat and you could see fishing lines and poles everywhere." He could see the legs and lower body of Olivieri. He resurfaced. Dunning again tried to coax Karen out of the cabin. She refused. Dunning now felt Olivieri was in imminent danger of drowning. He made the decision to enter the cabin. Dunning took a large breath and dived under. "As soon as I went in the door," said Dunning, "I went straight up and she was right next to me."

Surfacing within the cabin, Dunning found Olivieri trapped within a small two-by-two-foot air space, with the water up to her chest, and he immediately began calming her down while working to free her from fishing lines. Once he freed Karen of the lines, Dunning checked her for injuries and prepared for swimming out.

"He made me take my glasses off," Karen recalled, "and I can't see without my glasses at all. These are my lucky glasses, they didn't even fall off my face when I went into the water." Dunning placed the "lucky glasses" in his pocket, told Karen to hold onto the back of his leg, and, with her in tow, swam out to the surface. Once on the surface, they found themselves again tangled in fishing lines that threatened to pull them under. Other U.S. Coast Guard rescuers quickly came to their aid. It took Dunning three minutes to swim in and safely bring out Karen Olivieri. Karen and James had spent more than half an hour in the water. Back ashore, both received treatment for shock and hypothermia and were then released. Michael Dunning returned Karen's lucky glasses to her.

Michael L. Dunning received the Coast Guard Medal and the Association for Rescue at Sea's Gold Medal for his work. Later, at a ceremony honoring Dunning, a woman asked him, "Was it scary?" Dunning replied, "Not at the time, I was just thinking of saving that woman's life."

11 | Helicopters and Rescue Swimmers

By 1964, U.S. Coast Guard aviation was shifting to an air arm consisting mostly of helicopters, just as Frank Erickson had foreseen. The service's primary helicopter was the Sikorsky HH-52A Seaguard, which first entered the U.S. Coast Guard in January 1963. This aircraft was amphibious, possessed a "boat type hull," and was the service's medium-range aircraft. This does not mean it could land in heavy seas, however. It was also the first jet-powered helicopter in the U.S. Coast Guard. The HH-52A's great versatility proved its worth. When Hurricane Betsy struck the New Orleans, Louisiana, area in the autumn of 1965, U.S. Coast Guard pilots flying the HH-52A "rescued nearly 1,200 people" despite "constant threat from power lines, trees, structures and water." The last HH-52A helicopter retired from the service in 1989.[1]

In 1968, the service added the HH-3F Pelican to its inventory of rescue tools. Like the HH-52A, it could land on water. It also had a platform that could extend from the cabin door to help retrieve survivors. In October 1980, the HH-3F participated in the rescue of 320 passengers and 200 crew from the cruise ship *Prinsendam* in the Gulf of Alaska.[2]

The HH-65A Dolphin entered the service in 1985. Built by Aerospatiale Helicopter Corporation, a French firm with an assembly plant at Grand Prairie, Texas, the HH-65A is the service's short-range (248 miles) helicopter.[3]

The Sikorsky HH60J Jayhawk entered the service in December 1990, replacing the Pelican. Versions of this aircraft are in use today by the U.S. Army (the Black Hawk) and U.S. Navy (the Sea Hawk). The aircraft has a range of three hundred nautical miles and can transport a crew of four and a "maximum of six survivors from the maximum SAR radius." The aircraft is the service's medium-range SAR helicopter.[4]

By 1995, the two helicopters in SAR service within the U.S. Coast Guard were the HH-60J Jayhawk and the HH-65A Dolphin. Both helicopters have fine records within the service, but one thing they cannot do is set down on the sea, as could the HH-52A and HH-3F. This fact lead to a new feature in U.S. Coast Guard search and rescue work. To understand this development, it is necessary to examine a maritime event in 1983.

On Thursday evening, 10 February 1983, the *Marine Electric* sailed from Norfolk, Virginia, for Brayton Point, Massachusetts, carrying 25,000 tons of pulverized coal. The 13,757-gross-ton T-2-type bulk carrier shipped a crew of thirty-four. The next morning, the 587.5-foot *Marine Electric* battled seas estimated between twenty and forty feet, with winds screaming at sixty knots. Straining against the weather, the vessel took green water over her decks. At midnight, the captain had the holds checked to ensure the cargo was secure. Back came the frightening report that the sea was flooding into the holds.[5]

At 4:00 A.M. on Saturday, 12 February, the captain of *Marine Electric* ordered a radio call for help sent to the U.S. Coast Guard. By the time an HH-3F helicopter from Air Station Elizabeth City, North Carolina, arrived on scene, the ship had sunk and the crew were fighting for their lives in the frigid waters.

The pilot of the helicopter, Lt. Scott Olin, hovered over the men in the water. An attempt to use the rescue hoist proved fruitless; the sailors were too weak from hypothermia to grab the rescue basket. Lieutenant Olin immediately radioed that he needed assistance from a Navy helicopter with a rescue swimmer stationed at U.S. Naval Air Station Oceana, Virginia Beach, Virginia.

The Navy did not have a ready crew on the weekends and had to recall a pilot and crew. The Navy helicopter joined the U.S. Coast Guard helicopter on scene at 6:05 A.M. with U.S. Navy rescue swimmer Petty Officer James McCann on board the aircraft. McCann entered the forty-foot seas and swam until exhausted. The weather was so bad, McCann's face mask froze. Despite his Herculean efforts, he could only rescue three people; thirty-one sailors perished. McCann received the Navy and Marine Corps Medal for his heroic efforts.

The congressional House Merchant Marine and Fisheries Committee held hearings on the inability of the U.S. Coast Guard helicopters to rescue people in the water. Congress mandated, in the Coast Guard Authorization Act of 1984, that the "Commandant of the Coast Guard . . . establish a helicopter rescue swimmer program for the purpose of training Coast Guard personnel in rescue swimming skills."[6]

Originally the school for this skill was within the U.S. Navy, but in 1998 the program split from the Navy and is now at the U.S. Coast Guard Aviation Technical Training Center at Elizabeth City, North Carolina. The course of instruction is sixteen and a half weeks. A person entering this field must also attend a three-week emergency medical technician (EMT) school and be able to pass all the academic requirements to become an aviation life-support technician. Enlisted people assigned to this field are in the Aviation Survival Technician rating, previously known as Aviation Survivalman.[7]

While in a helicopter, the Aviation Survival Technician dresses in a wet or dry suit and carries a swimming facemask, fins, and snorkel. The swimmer also has a Tri-SAR harness, with signal flares, radio, knife, flashlight, and strobe light. Lastly, the rescue swimmer has an EMT kit.[8]

Rescue swimmers are now an important part of aviation search and rescue. Some of their work borders on the fantastic.

The sight of someone leaping out of a hovering helicopter into the sea, known within the service as a "free fall deployment," garbed in swim fins and mask, to rescue a survivor quickly captured the attention of the public and news media. Soon recruiting films and television shows featured rescue swimmers jumping, or being lowered, into stormy waters to help someone.

THE ONLY THING AHEAD WAS BLACK NIGHT

Lt. Cdr. John M. Lewis was the senior duty officer of U.S. Coast Guard Air Station, Corpus Christi, Texas, on Thursday, 15 April 1976. Lewis had entered the service in 1959 as an enlisted man and served in the aviation branch. For five years, he served as a radio and radar operator on fixed-wing aircraft. After graduating from Officer Candidate School and flight training in 1966, he flew fixed-wing aircraft. In 1974, Lewis learned to fly helicopters, and by 1976 he was flying both fixed-wing and rotary-wing aircraft. In short, on this Thursday, Lieutenant Commander Lewis was a seasoned U.S. Coast Guard aircraft pilot. He would soon have his skills tested.[9]

At 8:10 P.M. the station's radio watchstander contacted Commander Lewis and told him that he had "just received a phone call from a Marathon [oil company] representative . . . that an oil rig was sinking 20 miles out in the Gulf, with 50 people on board." Lewis pressed the SAR alarm and announced on the public address system, "Put both helicopters on the line." He gave orders to prepare the second helicopter for launching and to call the U.S. Navy, which was on the same airfield, to ask for their assistance. There was another U.S. Coast Guard helicopter crew from New Orleans at the station resting from a training flight. Lewis gave orders for that crew to stand by. After all this, he ran to the ready helicopter.

Eight minutes after receiving the call, Lieutenant Commander Lewis was climbing into the HH-52 helicopter, number 1444, and preparing to depart. Ens. John J. DiLeonardo, copilot—a Navy exchange pilot—and Aviation Machinist Mate 2d Class Harold J. Thomas Jr. flew with Lewis.

En route to the oil rig, moderate to severe turbulence shook the helicopter. Winds gusted to sixty knots, with seas cresting at twenty-five feet. The winds were so strong that it slowed the helicopter from its top speed of 109 knots to 50 knots. The large number of oil rigs in the area added to the difficulties of identifying which rig needed help.

Lewis eventually got in touch with the 166-foot rig, named *Ocean Express,* a "jack-up" rig (a drilling rig towed to a location). Once at a site, the rig lowers a "mat" to the ocean bottom. The mat has three cylindrical legs 12 feet in diameter and 312 feet in height. A hydraulic jacking system raises the three legs, which holds the drilling platform above the water. The three legs, arranged in a triangle, have one leg at the centerline of the bow of the rig and one each at the port and starboard corners. Lewis learned the correct position of the distress was forty miles out instead of twenty.[10]

Lewis opened radio contact with the captain of the rig, who said that the oil rig was not sinking but had taken "at least one large wave" that had loosened some pipes. Tugs were trying to steady the rig by holding it into the wind. Lewis asked if the captain wished to evacuate the people from the oil rig in case the situation worsened. The captain replied that that was what he wanted.

Meanwhile, Capt. Howard B. Thorsen, the station's commanding officer, came into the station to pilot the unit's second helicopter, the 1429. Years later, now Vice Admiral (Ret.) Thorsen recalled that it "didn't take long to get to the hangar, don my flight gear, and go out to the helo, which was already turning." He said the weather was so bad it felt "like the helo would take off on its own. As we got airborne, the air controller [on the] tower radio announced that all personnel were abandoning the tower, due to the winds."[11] Captain Thorsen flew a few miles and minutes behind Lewis.

Lewis, as he neared the position of *Ocean Express,* realized he might have to try a landing on the rig. The captain of the rig informed Lewis that "there was an obstruction 100 feet high just behind . . . [the landing pad]." As Lieutenant Commander Lewis approached the rig, he learned things were deteriorating rapidly. The captain of *Ocean Express* radioed the helicopter that he had put his crew into and launched escape capsules. Enclosed devices, the capsules had a small diesel engine and were designed not to roll over. They had only one escape hatch. The captain remained on the rig, "clinging to the railing, [and] communicating with a hand held radio."

Lewis approached the rig from its stern at eight hundred feet, with the wind coming across the rig's port bow. The whole rig had heeled over at least twenty degrees to starboard. As he approached for a basket pickup, he could see *Ocean Express* lit up and spotted the escape capsules in the water. Waves "were crashing over the rig," throwing spray high into the air. Later, Commander Lewis would remark, "I didn't really want to go down near that thing." The captain of *Ocean Express,* however, radioed "he was the last one," and he asked Lewis to pick him up. The captain made his way to the port side of the helicopter pad.

Lewis began his attempt at a pick up. "As I came down," he recalled, "my first thought was . . . to stay away from [the] legs which were jacked up maybe . . . a hundred feet. . . . I came in and tried to establish a hover." To establish the hover, Lewis needed a visual reference. When he tried to establish such a reference, everything in front of him was black, and with the turbulent sea, there was no horizon. In addition, the rig was canted at least twenty to twenty-five degrees. When Lewis looked at the rig, it caused him to experience "a type of vertigo." Adding to his problems, the helicopter shook with turbulence. Although his hoist operator tried to help him keep positioned through a steady flow of information through the intercom, Lewis had to pull the helicopter away from his approach.

As Lewis came around for another attempt, Captain Thorsen in the 1429 saw the rotating beacon of Lewis's helicopter and made for the scene. Thorsen recalled that Lewis radioed, "Captain, I don't think we can do this. There's no reference and it's too rough." Thorsen remembered the "jack-up rig had legs that, being retracted, were way up over the platform level, perhaps [eighty] or more feet. The only direction from which to make the approach meant that [Lewis] had to come in along the right side of the platform, and when he did so, he lost all visual reference to the entire rig. The only thing ahead of him was black night, swirling winds carrying varying quantities of waters and those legs were at his 8 o'clock position. . . . He dared not be anywhere near the left side of the platform or he was in danger of striking one of them with either a main or tail rotor blade . . . instant death for all on board."

Captain Thorsen's helicopter had a powerful searchlight, nicknamed "night sun." He maneuvered the 1429 to illuminate *Ocean Express.* Thorsen recalled that his helicopter hovered "at an altitude of somewhere around 150 feet, maybe 100 yards downwind of the rig. . . . Our million candles made it daylight on the rig. . . . Cables were flapping about, some sparks were flying; general disarray, with sliding 'pieces' of equipment or parts."

On this approach, Lewis decided to try a hover directly over the rig's captain. Lewis recalled that "as long as I had the captain in sight and some reference I was all right, but as soon as I would get to where I had to move out beyond the rig, the only reference I had [was a] tower . . . and it was laying over and moving quite a bit. So, I abandoned that approach, but time seemed to be of the essence now, so rather than climbing out I moved over to the side and we moved back . . . We had a little discussion, me and the crew, and tried to get a little better organized for this next approach in because it looked like the rig was maybe 45 degrees by this time . . . When . . . the waves . . . were hitting . . . [the tower] . . . some of the waves and spray were getting into the helicopter."

Lieutenant Commander Lewis began his third attempt at rescue. He told DiLeonardo to monitor a seventy-five-foot hover on the radar altimeter. Lewis told Thomas "to just start letting the basket down and to be sure that he had it down on the platform." Lewis would recall he gave this order "because I knew I couldn't stay there very long, it was too turbulent. I don't want to say that the helicopter was out of control[,] but when I got over there it was blowing so hard and it was so turbulent that it was, just about."

This time, as Lewis approached the rig, the hoist operator, Thomas, had the basket about half way down to the rig. Then Lewis again lost his reference. About this time, Lewis remembered, "the copilot told me that we were losing altitude rapidly and I saw the thing coming up underneath us. . . . I began climbing out, getting above it. We thought we were going down at the time." What was happening, however, was *Ocean Express* was tilting and sinking.

Captain Thorsen, in 1429, watched as the basket approached the rig's captain. "We clearly saw [the captain] jump at the basket, just as the helo started to move forward and away, but weren't certain, at first, if he had made it or had missed. Then, we saw him in the swinging basket, slowly moving toward the helo['s] belly." Lewis's helicopter "moved slowly forward and to the right, and just as it moved out of the illuminated area surrounding the rig, the rig began to tilt more and more slowly, inescapably over until the legs were totally under water. Cecil B. DeMille couldn't have staged a more dramatic show. Many of the lights continued to burn long after they were totally submerged, sparks flew and then stopped."

Lieutenant Commander Lewis would later admit the rescue was "more of snatch than a hoist." The first thing the rig captain asked was "if the crew was all right." Later, Lewis learned that one of the capsules had capsized and at least seventeen crewmen had been lost.

For their work on this stormy night, John M. Lewis received the Distinguished Flying Cross and John J. DiLeonardo and Harold J. Thomas Jr. received Air Medals.

SHE NEVER GAVE UP

On Tuesday morning, 3 January 1989, the SAR alarm at the U.S. Coast Guard Air Station Astoria, Oregon, echoed throughout the unit. Usually aircraft from the station answered cases dealing with commercial fishing vessels or recreational boaters. This alarm proved different. An Air National Guard F-4 fighter had experienced difficulties and spun out of control.[12] The pilot and weapons officer ejected an estimated thirty-five miles due west of Tillamook Bay, Oregon, to the south of Astoria.

As the duty helicopter crew prepared for flight, the engineering officer came into the SAR center and informed the duty officer that another helicopter, the 6516, was also ready. Lt. Cdr. William W. Peterson, although not on duty, volunteered to take the flight. Lt. (j.g.) William L. Harper volunteered to fly as copilot. The duty officer piped a flight crew for the 6516. Answering the call was Aviation Electronicsman 2d Class James Reese and Aviation Survivalman 3d Class Kelly Mogk, the rescue swimmer. The duty helicopter and the 6516 prepared to launch.

As Peterson prepared to take off in company with the duty helicopter, a message over the radio changed the case. A fuel control problem on one of the duty helicopter's engines caused it to return to the hangar, placing the rescue in the hands of Peterson and his crew. They lifted off at 10:59 A.M.

Shortly after Peterson departed, the station's jet aircraft, a Falcon, took off from the Astoria Station. The Falcon, though not able to pick up survivors, might locate electronic signals from the airmen in the water and provide an electronic beam for the helicopter's directional finder to follow. At nearly the same time, U.S. Coast Guard Air Facility at Newport, Oregon, some 170 miles to the south of the downed pilots, also launched a helicopter. Peterson knew that the weather prevented any search from the jet and that distance would stop the other helicopter from arriving when he came on scene. In other words, only Peterson and his crew could rescue the pilot and his weapons officer.

Peterson flew at 140 knots and at altitudes between fifty and one hundred feet. He flew partially overland and then, when within three nautical miles of the coast, encountered a one-hundred-foot overcast, with mist and rain, and winds of fifteen to twenty miles an hour—typical Pacific Northwest winter weather. Peterson briefed his crew en route. He informed Petty Officer Mogk that she might have to go into the water. The small size of the aircraft meant that if Mogk recovered both airmen, there was a chance she would have to be left in the water and be picked up by the helicopter from Newport. The helicopter from Newport, however, had not yet received rescue swimmers for their aircraft. Morgk replied that she was ready.

Kelly Mogk, twenty-one, from Seattle, Washington, entered the U.S. Coast Guard after graduating high school. At five feet six inches and 115 pounds, Mogk had not planned to be a rescue swimmer. In 1985, while she trained to be an aviation survivalman, the service began the rescue swimmer program. The U.S. Coast Guard required that all in her program become rescue swimmers. At the time Mogk prepared to enter the cold North Pacific waters after the downed pilot, she was the first woman to have graduated from the U.S. Navy's tough rescue swimmer program, a graduation Mogk attributed to "mental, not physical toughness." She also said that "she never gives up."[13] Events would prove her right.

As Lieutenant Commander Peterson and his crew approached the probable position of the two airmen, the helicopter flew into a hole in the weather. Dense fog encompassed the hole, with low clouds overhead. From their aircraft the aircrew looked down on sixteen-foot seas with a six-foot wind chop. The helicopter's low altitude and the state of the sea made it difficult to spot anyone in the water. Occasionally, those in maritime search and rescue receive a lucky break. Peterson glimpsed something white, like a white smoke signal, out of the right window. He quickly put the helicopter in a steep turn only to come upon a pod of spouting whales. As he turned to come back onto his base course, the helicopter flew over two small black rafts. Peterson later said finding the rafts "was really almost pure luck." Lieutenant Harper, however, thought it was "almost divine intervention."

Peterson put 6516 into a sharp turn and came into the wind near the rafts, flying the helicopter into a low hover over them. One raft was empty. 2d Lt. Michael Markstaller of the Air National Guard clung to the second raft. From the hovering helicopter, Markstaller appeared in bad shape. Peterson hovered low enough to see Markstaller's face. The pilot's "skin was dark, his stare vacant." Peterson knew he had only a short time to save him.

Mogk, at this time a two-year veteran of rescue swimming work, needed to immediately enter the water. As speed was essential, Mogk elected to enter the water quickly rather than wait to be lowered by the hoist. Rescue swimmers know there is a certain risk of injury from a free fall into the sea. Peterson and Mogk both understood this risk. Peterson hovered 6516 five to ten feet above the top of the wave crests, and Mogk, in her dry suit, flippers, and swim mask, leaped out.

Mogk swam quickly to Markstaller's side. She found the pilot hypothermic and barely conscious. Trying to keep Markstaller awake, Mogk said, "Hang on. You'll be all right. We're here. The chopper's right up there." Markstaller tried to speak. The roar of the hovering helicopter and the sound of the sea prevented any understanding. Mogk squeezed the pilot's hand. Markstaller returned the squeeze "real hard."[14]

Something was pulling on Markstaller. Looking through her swim mask under the green sea, Mogk saw his deployed parachute twenty feet below, its lines wrapped around his legs and chest. Later Mogk said it looked like "all one big spaghetti mess."[15] The parachute acted as a drogue, threatening to pull the pilot under. Mogk knew she had to get the parachute off the pilot. As she started to work on the fittings, she found the harness unlike anything she had trained with. The parachute's release fittings did not work. In what she later called a "minor delay," Morgk made her decision. Markstaller could not help himself. His left arm and leg hung limply in the sea. His right arm, locked firmly on the raft, seemed disjointed at the shoulder. Mogk took a deep breath and went underwater to cut the shrouds, which were wrapped around Markstaller's legs. At the first cut, the knife did not sever the line. Mogk knew that if she managed to cut the shrouds, it would just mean extra lines fanning underwater, with additional chances of entanglement. She had to undo each line.

Mogk surfaced and gulped air. She said a few words of encouragement to Markstaller, took another deep breath, held it, and dived. Meanwhile, hovering above them, Peterson kept the 6516 as close to Mogk and Markstaller as possible. He watched

Mogk working. "She was repeatedly diving and coming back up and trying to hold him up because he was being pulled under. I sort of felt useless."

Copilot Lieutenant Harper recalled, "Both [Mogk and Markstaller] were taking quite a beating from the sea and wind. He was moving real slowly. Bill Peterson voiced a couple of times a concern that he might die while we sat there and watched." As Mogk worked in the fifty-two-degree water, the helicopter from Newport arrived on scene. It began to search for the weapons officer from the jet. For the next twenty minutes Mogk continued her struggle, while the two helicopters and the Falcon remained overhead.

Mogk finally removed the last shroud line entangled around Markstaller's body. The five-foot, 115-pound Mogk now had to wrestle the 240-pound Markstaller to the rescue hoist. The semiconscious pilot kept a death grip on the raft. "Okay, I've got you now. Let go of the raft!" Mogk shouted over and over. In Marstaller's foggy mind the grip on the raft registered safety, or perhaps he was unable to hear Mogk over the roar of the helicopter and the seas. Marstaller did not respond. Mogk reached for her knife to puncture the raft. Just then, Markstaller released his grip. She gave the signal to Peterson for the pickup.

Petty Officer James Reese, at the helicopter's hoist and using the helicopter's intercom, guided the helicopter over Mogk and Markstaller. Mogk received the rescue collar and struggled to work it under the downed pilot's arms. She gave the signal to bring Markstaller up.

When Lieutenant Commander Peterson saw Markstaller's "blue skin and black lips," he made a difficult decision. He radioed the helicopter from Newport that he thought the survivor was close to death. He requested that the other helicopter pick up Mogk as he flew to the hospital in Astoria. The Newport helicopter could fly Mogk to the other raft.

Peterson increased the cabin heat in the helicopter and told Reese to break out the hypothermal warming bag. Reese over the intercom told Peterson that "this guy is really big. I don't think I can handle him. I need some help back here. He's badly hurt, too."

Peterson told his copilot, Lieutenant Harper, to make his way aft in the crowded helicopter and help Reese. As Harper struggled to release himself from belts and communications plugs, Reese said to Peterson, "This guy is really cold. Somebody's going to have to get in that bag with him. I'm too big. We both won't fit."

Once Markstaller was within the cabin, Harper and Reese found the pilot had a broken left arm and his right arm was dislocated at the shoulder. The quick examination revealed other injuries: his left leg had a ninety-degree bend between knee and ankle, while his boot, still fully laced, was dangling half off his left foot and was full of blood. Harper stripped to his underwear and got in the bag with Markstaller. Following advice from Commander Peterson, Harper kept up a constant stream of talk, trying to make Markstaller remain awake.

Mogk now floated alone. She was losing feeling in her hands and water had leaked into her dry suit. She knew she was fast approaching hypothermia. It took five minutes for the helicopter from Newport to pick up the rescue swimmer.

In the back of 6516, Harper and Reese worked on Markstaller. Peterson took over flying, navigation, and communications and turned toward Astoria, requesting a direct landing at the local hospital. As the helicopter sped northward, the Newport helicopter radioed that "your rescue swimmer just collapsed back here. She looks hypothermic. She's draining water. I don't see anything at the other raft. I don't recommend she go back down." Peterson radioed his agreement that Mogk should remain in the helicopter, but it was her decision. Mogk could not see the second flight officer and wisely felt she was in no condition to go back into the water. The Newport helicopter flew her to the Astoria Air Station, where she received treatment for hypothermia and a wrenched back from the hoist.

Peterson called with an estimated time of arrival at the hospital of twenty minutes. The hospital did not have a helicopter landing pad, which meant that Peterson had to land between light poles and parked cars. Fortunately, the hospital staff did not tarry while awaiting the helicopter. They had ordered special blood-warming equipment flown in from Portland and had moved cars for Peterson's landing. At the time of his admittance to the hospital, Marksteller's core temperature was only eighty-five degrees, on the borderline of unconsciousness. Marksteller recovered.

Peterson returned to the air station, refueled, picked up a new crew, then flew back to the datum buoy he had dropped when first spotting the rafts. He later recalled that he knew by returning to the location he would be a "guide dog" for other aircraft arriving to help.

The weapons officer, 1st Lt. Mark Baker, was found dead in a tangle underneath his raft. He had two broken arms, and "there was doubt whether he had even been conscious when he hit the water." The two airmen received their injuries when they ejected from their fighter at a speed considered too fast.

The best comment on the rescue effort came from Lieutenant Commander Peterson. Because of the death and weather, he said, "this mission was hard for . . . Kelly Mogk, who was on her first rescue. But I could remember that someone died on my first seven flights after I became a Coast Guard pilot. I thought, Am I a jinx? But in the twelve years since, I've saved many people on hundreds of search and rescue cases, and it's been very fulfilling. These were the worse conditions under which I've ever put a rescue swimmer down, and the effort Kelly Mogk made is what makes our work worthwhile."

For demonstrating "exceptional fortitude and daring despite extreme conditions that tested the limits of her endurance," Kelly Mogk received the Air Medal. William W. Peterson received the Coast Guard Commendation Medal, his second such award. He also received from the Oregon National Guard the Meritorious Service Medal.[16]

LET ME HAVE JUST ONE MORE

Bound from St. Augustine, Florida, to the Virgin Island, the 40-foot sailboat *Mirage* faced a strong weather system sweeping the eastern seaboard. The tyro sailors aboard the sailboat had little or no experience in the stormy Atlantic. Each day the wind increased and the seas built. Sleep was impossible. A frontal passage brought huge, thrashing seas, and the engine on board the sailboat quit.

On 23 January 1995, Allen Brugger, *Mirage*'s captain, took over the helm at dark. Three hours later, a series of fifty-foot waves slammed into the sailboat. *Mirage* rolled 120 degrees then righted itself. Everything on deck was swept away. The boat's violent motion flung crewman Mark Cole across the cabin, and he now had difficulty orienting himself. Two to three feet of water sloshed within the cabin, carrying with it food, cushions, and other debris. His orientation became more difficult as the cabin lights blinked out.

Cole fought his way out of the cabin. In the cockpit he saw only Captain Brugger. Crewman Fred Neilson was gone, washed overboard. Someone spotted Neilson, dragging in the wake, still attached to his safety harness. Another wave now ripped the life raft loose and it crashed overboard. The crew's hope for survival washed away. Brugger and Cole worked to pull in the panic-stricken Neilson to the relative safety of *Mirage*. Recovered, the badly shaken Neilson went below.

Inexperience continued to compound the problems. Crewman Dave Denman finally figured out how to operate the radio. No one knew how to operate the emergency position indicating radio beacon (EPIRB), nor did they know how to attach the antenna to the device.

At 8:30 P.M., U.S. Coast Guard units at Hampton Roads, Virginia, and Cape May, New Jersey, received a Mayday call on the international distress frequency. Denman had at last managed to get a message out. The boat was sinking, the life raft was gone, and those on board *Mirage* had lost all hope for rescue.

Some 320 miles to the northwest of the knocked-down *Mirage*, an HH-60J Jayhawk, number 6019, with Lt. Jay Balda as pilot, lifted off from U.S. Coast Guard Air Elizabeth City, North Carolina. On board as the duty rescue swimmer was Aviation Survivalman 1st Class Michael Odom. Earlier, U.S. Coast Guard

HC-130H, number 1502, Lt. Matt Reid, aircraft commander, had departed for the location of *Mirage*.

The faster HC-130H arrived on scene first. Lieutenant Balda knew he had enough fuel to remain on scene for approximately fifty minutes. Reid in the HC-130H talked to *Mirage* via radio and began the preparation for the rescue hoist so the Jayhawk would not waste time upon arrival at the sailboat's position.

The first of many problems that would take place on this storm-tossed night began a little after the HC-130H arrived in the area. Reid radioed Balda that Brugger refused their offer of dropable pumps and survival kits. Brugger informed Reid that the sailboat was taking on water from an unknown source. The helicopter crew discussed their rescue tactics on the flight to the sailboat and decided the best course of action was to put a rescue swimmer into the water. The seas were too rough for a novice to attempt getting into the rescue basket by himself. First, the sailboat would stream a line behind their boat. Odom, the rescue swimmer, would hold onto the line. Then a crewman from *Mirage* would leap into the water. Odom, holding onto the line, would grab the man and help him into the rescue basket. When both were in the basket, hoisting could begin. Once safely on board the Jayhawk, the rescue helicopter's crew repeated the cycle until all in *Mirage* reached safety. This type of maneuver had worked in the past, though the tactic did presume that a boat had no speed other than the action of the seas and wind.

Reid in the circling fixed-wing aircraft passed the plan onto the men in the sailboat. The pilot also did a prehoist checklist before the arrival of the Jayhawk, insuring the operation could begin when the slower-moving helicopter arrived.

The Jayhawk flew over *Mirage* at 1:10 A.M. As instructed, the sailboat crew streamed a line some fifty feet long from the stern, with a boat fender tied to the seaward end. Yet another problem arose. For some unknown reason, Brugger kept up *Mirage*'s sails. This meant a pickup attempt while in pursuit of the sailboat. Brugger radioed his refusal to leave the sailboat. The U.S. Coast

Guard's Rescue Coordination Center (RCC) radioed that the "helo [would] rescue all of them or none."[17]

The message to *Mirage* from RCC caused some confusion in the helicopter. Were they to pick up the sailboat's crew? Balda moved the Jayhawk away from the sailboat. The helicopter crew now received an unwanted surprise. Thirty seconds after the men on board *Mirage* received the remain on board message from RCC, Mark Cole leaped into the water. Once in the sea, Cole's cold hands could not hold onto the line trailing from the sailboat due to the boat's speed. He slipped away from his lifeline.

Odom, sitting in the cabin door of the helicopter, dressed in his dry suit, swim fins, and swim mask, watched Cole in disbelief. Lieutenant Balda made a tight turn into the wind and dropped into a hover, all the while keeping sight of Cole. Odom was quickly lowered into the water with the end of the hoist cable snapped to his harness. Once into the cold, churning sea, he released the cable and swam toward Cole. The hoist operator brought the cable back on board the helicopter and attached it to the rescue basket, ready for lowering when Odom signaled he had Cole ready for pickup.

Cole's fear approached panic. He felt Odom touch him. "It was a great feeling when that fellow put his arm around me," Cole recalled. Grasping Cole, Odom began the difficult swim toward the helicopter. Lieutenant Balda, meanwhile, had trouble hovering. He had no visual references to hold position. Even if the helicopter was motionless, the sea gave a false sense of movement. Thirty-five to forty knots of wind tried to push the 6019 away from Odom and Cole.

Aviation Machinist Mate 3d Class Mark Bafetti, flight mechanic and hoist operator, leaned out the helicopter's side door. Held in by his safety strap, Bafetti was able to guide Balda over Odom and Cole. Over the internal communications system (ICS), Bafetti said, "Back ten—right, back, back—hold, hold, hold—left five—stop, hold." Bafetti guided the basket downward with his left hand while he controlled the up and down movement with a push button controller in his right. Slack in the cable might loop around a person in the water and then tighten, seriously injuring or killing the person. Odom just touched the basket, only to have a wave suddenly drop him, jerking the basket away.

Balda and Bafetti continued their attempts. Odom finally grabbed the basket and stuffed Cole into it. In panic, Cole froze and refused to sit. His head and shoulders rose above the basket bail. Cole wrapped his arms around the bail placing his head, arms, and torso next to the whipping cable. A wave passed, jerking the basket out of the water. Yet Cole somehow remained in the basket, which again landed in the water. Odom swam hard to the basket to check out Cole, who appeared uninjured. The basket again started up, swinging wildly, with the cable striking the helicopter. After twenty minutes of struggle, Bafetti brought Cole safely on board the helicopter, but four more people remained in the sail-boat and only thirty minutes of fuel remained. Next, Odom came on board. Balda quickly turned the helicopter in pursuit of *Mirage,* now nearly a mile away.

Thomas Steier was next to leap into the sea from *Mirage.* Odom, again, in the sea and hanging onto the trailing line, prepared to capture the frightened novice sailor. The rescue swimmer grabbed Steier and said, "Hey, as long as I got you nothing's going to happen to you, and I'm taking care of you and don't worry about it." Steier, at six feet two inches tall, had difficulty getting into the basket in the crashing seas. Finally, Odom gave the signal to Bafetti to hoist. Ten feet into the air, a large wave engulfed Steier. The basket snapped and swung in circles when released from the wave, striking the bottom of the helicopter and fuel tank. The hoist operator pulled the rescue basket into the helicopter's cabin.

Odom later remembered that the wave that buried Steier "scared the heck out of me to the point where I was swimming like heck to get out of the way of the aircraft. I've never seen water so close to a helicopter. . . . [Bafetti] jumped back in the aircraft and dropped his hoist unit and backed off." The wave did not strike the 6019, and Bafetti lowered the hoist and picked up Odom. The wave "was a good twenty-five to thirty-five footer." Odom and Lieutenant Balda agreed that the next hover should be at a higher altitude.

The backup rescue swimmer, Aviation Survivalman 3d Class Michael Vittone, helping in the back of the helicopter, worried about Odom's fatigue. Vittone said, "Are you ready for me to go, Mike?" Odom replied, "One more. Let me have just one more." It had taken nearly forty minutes to recover only two survivors. Time and fuel were running out. Three more survivors waited on board *Mirage*.

Balda again brought his helicopter to the sailboat and Odom entered the water. This time he hit the sea very hard. Gasping for air, he sucked in seawater and vomited. Nevertheless, he swam to the rope and grabbed the next person, who leaped into the water. Odom, still vomiting, positioned himself and the survivor underneath the helicopter, now hovering at one hundred feet above them. Bafetti had difficulty keeping the slack out of the cable and avoiding the high seas. The survivor clambered into the basket and hoisting began. Vittone lay on the deck of the helicopter's cabin using both hands to help keep the cable away from the aircraft. The basket continued to swing in wide circles as it ascended. The arcing cable slammed into "the 120-gallon fuel tank that hung from the right side of the aircraft. Next, the cable slid along the cabin's door frame, flew out hitting the side of the tank, and then repeated the arc."

Vittone felt spurs of wire from the cable. He yelled to Bafetti. By now the survivor was sixty to seventy feet in the air. Bafetti ran the hoist at full speed, hoping to get the hoist finished before the cable snapped. He succeeded.

Lt. (j.g.) Guy Pearce, the copilot, said over the ICS, "Six minutes to bingo." Six minutes of time remained before the helicopter had to depart. Time now made it impossible to recover Odom. Bafetti tried signaling Odom with his flashlight to call on his radio. Odom did not answer. The pilot flashed his hover lights, meaning he had lost sight of the rescue swimmer. It is the only signal to the swimmer there is a problem. Odom, thinking the crew of 6019 had lost sight of him, fired a flare and attached a strobe light to the top of his head. The copilot called out, "Bingo."

The bewildered Odom watched as the rescue basket dropped into the sea. The 6019 hovered about two hundred yards away. Odom saw the datum marker buoy go into the water. "I looked at that and it didn't look right," he recalled. He knew something was wrong. Odom could not understand why the crew of the 6019 could not see him. The Jayhawk moved slowly over him.

Now seven minutes over the fuel exhaustion time, the 6019 crew made their final preparations to leave Odom. Vittone kicked out a life raft and closed the helicopter's door. The life raft landed within arm's reach of Odom. The helicopter departed the area, leaving Odom in the dark fighting the high seas. Odom screamed into his radio: "Nineteen talk to me! What's going on? Nineteen talk to me!" Odom could not receive 6019's transmissions because both were trying to talk at the same time, blocking each other out.

Survivor Steier, shivering in the rear of the helicopter, was not aware of what was going on. He knew two men remained on *Mirage* and Odom was in the water. The cabin door closed. "We had no idea what's going on," he said. "I looked over at [Vittone] . . . and he had tears in his eyes. And I didn't have any idea what in the world was goin' on."

Odom clambered on board the life raft, but before he could attach a lanyard to himself and the raft, waves hurled him back into the cold sea. Odom swam back, slid into the raft, and attached the lanyard. Exhausted, he felt the first stages of panic. The only thing in his immediate area was the HC-130H circling high overhead.

In the C-130, pilot Lieutenant Reid, now on scene for nearly four hours, also faced the inevitable fuel problem. He received radioed orders to return to base. The crew of C-130, number 1502, however, refused to leave Odom alone in the dark. A relief C-130 would not arrive until the fuel tanks in 1502 were empty. Reid, defying orders, shut down two of the aircraft's four engines, conserving his remaining fuel.

Odom was very sick on the raft. Seasickness and depression further weakened him. There were no ships or aircraft nearby that could help, even though diverted U.S. Navy and merchant ships were steaming toward the area. The two Jayhawks at Elizabeth

City that might help him were out of commission in the hangar. Lt. Mark Russell, the copilot in the orbiting 1502, attempted to bolster Odom with encouragement. He told the rescue swimmer another plane was on the way, although it would be over an hour before anything could even take off. The crew of 1502 began to drop flares.

The encouragement and human voice helped. Odom later recalled that the two U.S. Coast Guardsmen started bantering a bit. Over the radio they recalled a rumored incident when an aircraft dropped a flare that accidentally landed in a raft of Cubans. Odom said to Russell, "Remember, I'm not a Cuban."

Another wave crashed into the raft, flinging Odom back into the sea. His lanyard kept him tethered to the raft and once more he clambered into relative safety. Panic again seized him. He called out that he needed help fast. Odom was constantly on his knees in the raft with dry heaves. Lieutenant Russell suggested Odom open the emergency survival pack and drink fresh water. Odom, however, could not open it. He started to pull out his survival knife but realized he might puncture the raft. He removed his survival glove to untie the line closing the survival pack, but the sea took the glove. He finally got the package containing the water, tore it open with his teeth, and drank it. He immediately regurgitated.

Soon, Odom was suffering from stomach cramps. Lieutenant Russell was now busy helping the pilot fly the aircraft and handling communications between the aircraft and Miami and Elizabeth City. Aviation Machinist Mate 1st Class Barry Freeman, the flight mechanic, took over the communications with Odom. Freeman continued a flow of encouragement to the weakening rescue swimmer.

Odom was rapidly slipping away to unconsciousness. As his body temperature fell, he could no longer lift the small handheld radio and he had trouble focusing his eyes. He tried to keep an eye on the low-flying C-130. At this point, he lost all hope for rescue and prepared for death. He managed to lash himself face up in the raft, so they could find his body.

As Odom awaited death, crews at Elizabeth City worked feverishly to get the second HC-130 ready. Other mechanics repaired Jayhawk number 6034. Regulations required a daytime test flight after repairing a helicopter. The air station commander, Capt. Stanley J. Walz, waived this regulation.

Lt. Cdr. Bruce Jones and his Jayhawk crew departed as soon as his aircraft was ready. Jones flew at seven thousand feet to conserve fuel. During the flight, the helicopter encountered ice, so Jones brought the helicopter to a lower altitude, lost the ice, and continued with his mission. In the meantime, the relief HC-130 arrived over Odom. Lt. Cdr. Dan Osborn, the pilot of the aircraft, helped guide Jones in the helicopter to the scene. The merchant ship *Diletta F* arrived as daybreak started dimly lighting the area. The ship could not rescue Odom but could provide some shield from the wind and seas for the rescue helicopter.

Lieutenant Commander Jones started his helicopter into a hover over Odom at 6:13 A.M., four hours and fifty minutes after Odom went into the water. Over an hour had passed since Odom transmitted his last words, "I'm cold, I'm cold."

The rescue swimmer on board the 6034, Aviation Survivalman 3d Class Jim Peterson, was lowered into the raft. Straddling Odom, Peterson shouted and rubbed the apparently lifeless Odom. As Peterson reached under Odom's survival hood for a pulse, Odom's arm reached into the air. Quickly Peterson snapped Odom's harness to his harness and signaled for the hoist. Peterson's arm became entangled in the webbing of the life raft. The water-filled raft placed great strain on the hoist cable. A few tugs freed the raft, and Odom reached the safety of the helicopter.

Many miles away, *Mirage* still moved ahead with two people on board. An HC-130 from the Clearwater Air Station, Florida, orbited over the sailboat. Lieutenant Commander Jones, in the Jayhawk that had just recovered Odom, received radioed orders from RCC to proceed to the sailboat and hoist the remaining two men. Jones reported that Odom was in critical condition and needed immediate medical attention. This changed the situation. Jones now had to bring the rescue swimmer to a hospital at least two hours away. Jones opted to divert to the U.S. Navy's *Ticonderoga,* steaming toward the scene and 150 miles away. He felt he could drop off Odom for immediate attention, refuel on board the ship, and then go to *Mirage.*

The aircrew of the Jayhawk found Odom's body temperature was 92.5 degrees. The crew in the back of the helicopter cut off Odom's survival gear, wrapped him in blankets, and started him on oxygen. The pilots turned the heat in the cabin to its highest setting. During the one-hour-and-ten-minute flight to the *Ticonderoga,* Odom's body temperature climbed to 97.1 degrees. On board the Navy ship, corpsmen started medical work on Odom immediately after they received him in sick bay. His recovery was rapid, but he remained in sick bay for twenty-four hours.

The two crewmen on board *Mirage* were still claiming they were in distress and wanted helicopter evacuation. After refueling the Jayhawk on the aircraft carrier, Lieutenant Commander Jones proceeded to the sailboat. One of the crewmen left the boat and was quickly picked up. *Mirage*'s captain, Brugger, still refused to leave. Jones informed Brugger that he was departing with the survivor.

The following day, Odom was flown from the *Ticonderoga* to U.S. Marine Corps Air Station Cherry Point, North Carolina, where he was picked up by his station's aircraft for a welcoming home. Odom returned to work the next day, and three days later he was again in a helicopter on another rescue mission. For his efforts on the *Mirage* rescue, Michael Odom received the Distinguished Flying Cross.

Brugger sailed on after the U.S. Coast Guard's aircraft departed and arrived at his destination at St. Thomas, Virgin Islands, after a seventeen-day passage. Here, he prepared *Mirage* for winter charter service.

12 | Station Yaquina Bay, Oregon

For the most part, those who serve at the U.S. Coast Guard's small boat rescue stations are virtually anonymous. They do their duty with pride and perform brave deeds, yet the public knows little about them. But one station, Yaquina Bay at the central Oregon coastal city of Newport, is the home station to two men who overcame the anonymity.

Like most of the harbors along the rugged Pacific Northwest coast, the passage into Newport Harbor is over a bar. Chief Warrant Officer John Dodd, former commanding officer of Station Yaquina Bay, said that the bar "is one of the last . . . to close when heavy weather hits. I have sat out on the bar with very steep 18- to 20-foot swells rolling through and they do not break. So we can conduct many 'rough bar standbys' as the fishermen work at getting back into port. However, once the bar decides to break, it will break 18 to 25 feet and it will be about three to five rows deep. Very nasty."[1]

THOMAS D. McADAMS

Master Chief Thomas D. McAdams is arguably the most famous U.S. Coast Guard enlisted man on record. He has appeared in *Life*,

National Geographic, True, and other national magazines. CBS's Charles Kuralt featured the master chief on network television. A motor lifeboat with McAdams at the wheel even made an episode of the television series *Lassie.* One old salt told a historian that after the show aired, there were many times when McAdams answered the telephone only to hear the caller say, "Woof! Woof!" and hang up.[2]

McAdams earned the reputation of being the service's best boatman. His major military decorations include the Legion of Merit (one of the very few U.S. Coast Guard enlisted men to receive this award), the Coast Guard Medal, Gold Life Saving Medal, Coast Guard Achievement Medal, Coast Guard Commendation Medal, Coast Guard Unit Commendation Ribbon, and other decorations. His civilian awards include an Oregon Governors Award, the City of Newport, Oregon, Valor Award, and the Newport Chamber of Commerce Award for Civil Achievement.

When McAdams came into the U.S. Coast Guard in 1950, the 36-foot motor lifeboat was the mainstay of the small boat stations, and he remained on active duty long enough to work with the designing of the service's new 47-foot motor lifeboat. He joined the service when small crews were the norm and spent most of his career in a limited geographical area, much like the keepers of the U.S. Life-Saving Service.

Sailors carry two seabags—one imaginary, full of stories, which they will bring out at a moment's notice. There are sea storytellers and there are sea storytellers that make an art of the tradition. McAdams is also a master chief of storytellers. Sit for a few minutes and watch his hands gesturing, making the movements of a pitching, rolling motor lifeboat. Listen to his voice rising to a crescendo at the proper places and, even if you have never been to sea, you will know you are in the presence of a natural sea storyteller.

McAdams developed two distinctive trademarks: one was a modified pilot's helmet he wore while on a lifeboat to both protect his head and to keep his "ears warm," the other was an ever-present cigar. The cigar became a part of the mythology that grew up around the master chief, something that McAdams did little to scotch. Charles Kuralt learned the standard refrain heard up and down the coast: "As long as the cigar is lit, you can relax. But when it begins to get soggy, that's when you have to pay attention. If he takes the cigar out, turns it around and sticks the lit end in his mouth, then you know you're going to get wet. But if you ever see him spit it out, then you better take a deep breath because you'll have to hold it a long time as the boat rolls over." There are very few, if any, photographs of McAdams on his motor lifeboat without his cigar.

McAdams began his career at the Yaquina Bay Station. He made chief petty officer at the unit and retired as officer in charge of the station in 1977. A reporter once described him as resembling "the actor Jimmy Cagney in looks, stance and staccato" speech. He enlisted in the U.S. Coast Guard on 7 December 1950, in Seattle, Washington, attended boot camp at Alameda, California, and then received orders to the U.S. Coast Guard's Thirteenth District. After a short stay at a base in Seattle awaiting assignment, he and three others received orders to the lifeboat station at Yaquina Bay.

After McAdams and the other new crewmen checked in, they received the night off. The four young men made their way to a local watering hole, the Pip Tide. Some fishermen ordered beers for the newcomers. One of the salts said, "So, you're going up there [to the station] and be with old 'Fancy Pants.'"

"What do you mean?" they asked.

"*You'll* find out!"

Years later, McAdams related that his first commanding officer was a warrant officer. He pointed out that at that time "a warrant officer to a seaman apprentice out of boot camp is God. At least one of his disciples. The commanding officer received the nickname 'Fancy Pants,' because he always wore his uniform and was straight-laced. If he drove downtown in his car and you were on the street, you'd better salute him." Unlike other warrant officers of the time, McAdams noted, Fancy Pants had no experience in small boats. The commanding officer was able to cover up his lack of experience by his talk. He also pretended that he was salty. As McAdams tells it, "If you went out in a lifeboat and got sea-sick—he never went out to sea in a lifeboat—one of the questions he would ask when you came back in with the lifeboat was who got seasick? He would then say, 'I want them to make every call until they get over seasickness.'"

When McAdams and the three other men reported to Yaquina Bay, the number of men at the unit increased to sixteen. The crew felt they were very lucky to have so many crewmen. Most of the boat training was on the job; duty was for eight days, twenty-four hours a day, and then two days off.

Besides the training on the motor lifeboats, five days a week the crew had other training in the basement of the station. This included practice in Morse code, wig-wag signals, semaphore, and knots. Much of the information came from a small blue book, *Manual for Lifeboatmen.* written for anyone assigned to a station.

McAdams recalled, "The CO was a stickler for training. He knew nothing about actual sea duty and small boats and the mis-ery of going to sea in the small boats, but he was a stickler for training. You had to learn the blue book and you had to learn it by heart. We didn't have a chief petty officer at the time. What you had was a man in a chief's uniform, but the pins were different: he was a surfman. We called him chief, but he was officially called 'number 1.'" This was a holdover from the old U.S. Life-Saving Service days when ranks were by numbers. The man who held the number 1 position would be second in command.

Today most people at the stations when they are ready to go on liberty ask the officer of the day if they can go ashore. At Yaquina Bay in the early 1950s, the procedure was quite different. If it was your turn to have your two days off, the crewman walked into the number 1's office at 10:00 A.M. and requested to attend complaint and request mast. The second in command would ask, "What's it about?" The crewman then responded with the request to see the commanding officer about having his two days off.

Number 1 checked his records. At the time, people on watch in the lookout tower periodically inserted a key, known as making a punch, into a watchman's clock to prove they were awake. If the watchstander missed a punch or was more than fifteen minutes late in making a punch, the crewmen did not even make it into the commanding officer's office and did not have time off duty.

If the crewman's record was clear, he entered the commanding officer's office. "You'd stand at attention," recalled McAdams. "The old man would shuffle papers while you stood there for a minute or two minutes, just to leave you standing at attention with your hat under your arm, in your dungarees. He'd look up and say, 'What is it?' You'd give your name, rate, and serial number and say, 'Request liberty, sir. This is the day of my liberty.'

"He'd check the sheet and say, 'Very well, you meet all requirements. You haven't missed any punches in the tower, that's very good. We have no complaints against you on your work and your drills. This week is distress signals. Give me number three and number eight from the book.' You'd better repeat them by heart. If you could, he'd say, 'Very well, you have permission to go on liberty.'

"If you could not recite it, he'd say, 'Come back and see me. I'm going home at sixteen hundred [4:00 P.M.] this afternoon. See the Number One and tell him you will be in here at sixteen hundred.' Then the rest of the afternoon you could go study the book. You didn't have to go back to work. You went up and studied until you knew it by heart. At sixteen hundred, you'd come back and recite it by heart. If you didn't, he'd say, 'Tomorrow at request and complaint mast.' Well, you'd already lost twenty-four hours of your liberty, so'd you go back and study.

"So you had to learn signals and then there was the beach cart. You had to learn all the numbers, the assignments for each of the crew's position in the beach cart drill. 'What's your number in the beach cart?' I'm number six, sir. You had to recite the duties of your number and the one aft of you. If there was no one aft of you, then you had to repeat the one forward of you."

The next commanding officer McAdams had at Yaquina Bay was "Mr. Harold Lawrence." McAdams remember that Warrant Officer Lawrence was an experienced lifeboatman and "one of the men I always looked up to." Many years later, McAdams met

Lawrence at a reunion, and, McAdams said, "he was still Mr. Lawrence to me. His teaching was great. He would tell stories. Sit at the table and tell sea stories. I would pick up things from those that I would use later. I would incorporate them into the motor lifeboat school when I took over and they became part of the procedures."

McAdams next served at the Coos Bay Station in Oregon and then went to a cutter. There, he received orders to Yaquina Bay again, this time as a boatswain's mate first class. "You know, the dividing line between glory and losing a stripe is very thin. I found this out on my second time at Yaquina Bay. In 1956, we got the 52-foot motor lifeboat here at Yaquina Bay. Whole new concept in boat handling. Twin screws single rudder. Whole new concept, but, boy, does it work.

"On this day in June 1957, everybody had a boat call and all the boats were out. It was foggy. The bar was good. A little swell. I'd just towed in a boat. I was back to the bell buoy, not even to the whistle buoy, when the tower called me and said, 'I have a boat. I can just see it through the fog and he is coming over the north reef.'

"The tower says, 'He's inside the reef! He's inside the reef!'

"By the time I got to the reef, the tower says, 'He's capsized! He's capsized! I have four people in the water! I think there's a dog there, too.' The tower watch is looking right down on it. So, we came across the reef. I knew the holes in the reef. You gotta know your rocks and holes. I came right on through.

"The people in the water were still fifty to one hundred yards ahead of me. I'm going to hit bottom. The 52-footer draws six feet aft and three feet forward. We hit bottom. Boom! The boat hit. I said, 'Oh, shit!'

"Here comes the next breaker. I waited until it picked me up and I turned the boat broadside. Surfed on the wave. I would ride on the wave broadside and come down on the side and put the people in the water in the lee of the boat.

"Boom!"

"I took the 52-footer right up to their small boat. But by this time the people were being carried away by the seas. There were two women and two men."

Pilots are not the only people who gesture with their hands when speaking about their exploits. Watch a lifeboat sailor sometime. As McAdams spoke, his hands showed the movements of a pitching, rolling motor lifeboat so much so that you could almost believe you could get seasick.

"In those days we did not have the restrictions on wearing lifejackets that we do today," McAdams continued. "None of us on the 52-footer had lifejackets on. I always considered myself an excellent swimmer. The people in the water had no lifejackets on.

"We hit bottom. I said, 'Grab those two people forward!'

"It was a man and his wife. He was in good shape, but he was holding his wife up. They were, I don't know, twenty or thirty feet from the boat.

"I said, 'I'll get them!' I ran across the lifeboat and dove completely over their boat that was upside down alongside of us. I hit the surf. Boom! Boom! I swam up to the guy.

"'How you doing?'

"'Okay, but my wife.' Her head was draggin' in the water. I started to swim them back to the lifeboat. You can go twenty or thirty feet towing somebody kickin'. I got them to the 52-footer's lifelines that hang over the side. I grabbed him and stuffed him in the lifeline and he's holding his wife. Then I crawled up onto the motor lifeboat. We're being smashed against the other boat. The breakers are coming over the boat. They weren't real big at that time because I'm inside the reef. So I climbed back upon the boat. I hear, 'Helllp!'

"This other guy, he's in bad shape. The woman he's got is floating away from him. He can't handle it anymore. There were four of us as crew on the lifeboat. I turned to one of the guys, name was Dean, James. 'Go get 'em!' Then, 'No, you get a lifejacket on!' I'm responsible for him. I got the lifejacket on him in a hurry. I gave him a shove and overboard he went.

"The guy was hanging on the lifelines forward, but Dean went and got the woman. He's coming back to the boat with her.

"Meanwhile, now there's three of us and we go get the guy in the lifeline. We drag this guy, onto the deck. God! He's two hundred some pounds. We get him on deck and he's breathing. So, I tied him onto the towing bit.

"By this time Dean is back with the woman, so we grab the woman.

"The guy aft, meanwhile, is going under everytime the boat goes down in the breakers. An' his wife is going under, too. He's losin' all his strength. We grab the woman and we pull the woman on board. I think she was almost out of it by this time. Barely breathing. I told my guy, 'Start artificial respiration.' In those days we used the back pressure arm lift method. He starts working on her a little bit. Then I go back and get the woman from this other guy.

"I now got one guy in the water, one guy working artificial respiration and so two of us go back to get this other woman. My crewman was the first colored guy at this station. Big guy. Good man. Good seaman. We really have to pull. On deck, she needs help. I yell, 'Start on her! Start on her!'

"The other woman's moaning and groaning. So the crewman comes over. We tie her in the towing bit. Then we go for the guy. All this time we're being hit broadside and being driven in. Well, it had been foggy. Here is where you talk about your fine line of getting a medal or losing a stripe. Either you're falling in glory or you're falling in shit.

"We get the guy back up on board. The woman starts to breath. We got the four people aboard. I said, 'Get them down below!'

"Now we're all going to be saved, but we're going to be washed upon the beach. Everybody's alive. Even the little dog. The dog had been swimming in circles and the guys from the beach party have him on the jetty. We got the four people locked down below.

"The fog had burned off in the middle of this operation. We are in bright sunlight. All of this had been going out over our radio. It's an old AM radio and the locals could all hear it. Cars coming across the bridge on Highway 101 were stopped and watching. The bridge was packed. We got hundreds watching this operation of the Coast Guard. They don't know what we're doing. All they see is a boat in the surf and people being pulled up on board and water breaking over the boat.

"The 36-footer from the station is just outside of us. The reef is now breaking pretty good. The 36-footer can't get to us, but they're going to try."

Using his twin screws and rudder, McAdams managed to work the 52-foot motor lifeboat off the beach but damaged the rudder. "The station at that time was run by an E-8 chief," he said. "The group was also here, with two warrant officers in charge. The chief was gone, but he got back while all this was happening. The group commander just chewed his ass out. 'That boat should not be in there! What's he doing with that boat in there? We're going to rake his ass! We're going to give you a letter of reprimand!'

"We've done a neat rescue. We've saved four lives. The crew down on the jetty saved a doggie. You should feel pretty good. Jesus! Everyone's getting an ass chewing!

"We had a real good engineer at the station. I said, 'What's the problem with the steering?' The steering was all by cable and when the rudder hit the bottom, it tore all the cable out. The engineer said he could run down to the store and, hell, for less than twenty dollars he had new brackets and in less than an hour he came up and said, 'She's ready to go.'

"I said, 'Okay, I'll be down. We got to get her out. We're still running calls.'

"The group called the chief back in again. Now, the boat's all right. God! There's twenty-five dollars damage. The warrant officer said to the chief, 'You'll tell him not to do that again! Stay away from the surf!' and on and on. Finally, the chief can't take this anymore and he wrote me a note and left the station.

"When I came in a couple of hours later, things had quieted down, most of the boats were in. I find the chief's note: 'Really sorry to leave you with this mess, but I had to get out of here or I would say something that would jeopardize my career.'

"One of the warrant officers in the group was a great old man. He didn't care, but he was a little nervous on this. The other guy was really. . . . I walked into the office and I told him, 'You gonna transfer me outta here? You'd better do it right now. If I get another call in the surf in the next five minutes I'm taking that boat in there. I don't give a damn if you don't like it. Far as I'm concerned, lives are more important than property. I won't abuse property, but I will use it to save lives. Not only that, I'll get ahold of the news media. I'm going to tell them exactly what you told the chief after we saved these lives. I'm going to tell them everything you said to the chief. You're not going to be talking to me. You're going to be talkin' to the whole damned public!'

"'Well, wait a minute! Before you do that, let's wait until tomorrow and we'll get the chief and we'll all have a nice talk. Settle down!'

"'All right. You give him any crap over this call and it comes back to me. I'm the guy that made the decision. I'm going to let everyone in the world know.'

"That ended it for the night. The next day is Monday. They make up a message. Had to make up a grounding report and this and that. Saved four lives, saved this, saved that. They really downplayed it. It was just nothing.

"Well, one of the people watching from the bridge was high up in the governor's office. The head captain of the Oregon State Patrol was also watching. Lot of visitors. The next morning they're writing letters and calling the district admiral. I never seen such a brave thing. The boat in the breakers. Guys diving over the side. They ought to get medals.

"The admiral's gettin' all these calls. All he's got is this little message. Then the governor's office calls and wants to congratulate the Coast Guard. The admiral calls his aide and says, 'You call the damn group down there and find out what in the hell is going on!'

"When the group finds out the admiral is asking about the rescue they say, 'Yes, we're going' to hang those guys.'

"'Hang those guys? We're going to give them medals! Jesus Christ!'

"Two of us got Gold Life Saving Medals and two got Silver Life Saving Medals. That's a fine line you walk. If the fog hadn't lifted I'd probably been busted."

At this time, before the Coast Guard Medal was authorized, the Gold and Silver Life Saving Medals were the two highest medals in peacetime U.S. Coast Guard personnel at small boat stations could receive. The awards board ruled McAdams's feat deserved to be called extraordinary heroism, and he received an extra 10 percent in his retirement pay.

McAdam's next transfer took him to an 83-foot patrol boat, which soon was decommissioned, and he took command of an 82-foot patrol boat. He then received orders to command the station at Cape Disappointment, Washington. "When I had the stations," he said, "I trained most of the people to be boat people. I went through people pretty quickly. I could weed out people. As in any job, there are a lot of people who just ride, they're hiding, staying back riding it out. They do their job, but they don't get into it. Same way in the fire department, you got the guys that really go in and hit the fires and then you got the others. You need those people to get the gear. They're not really into it."

Master Chief McAdams recounted one incident at Cape Disappointment Station that has vividly remained in his memory. There were so many deaths on one day that he "turned the garage into a morgue. It was a Sunday and in the little town of Ilwaco the guy from the funeral parlor was gone for the day, so I had to put the bodies in the garage. One woman calls in and she's all balled up. Her husband's missing. She gives a description of the boat he was in. 'Well, ma'am,' I said, 'we've had a lot of bad accidents today. I believe your husband's boat capsized and I believe we've got him.'

"'Oh, my God,' she says.

"'We don't have any identification on him. Do you have friends that can come into the station to identify him?'

"She said no. She came out herself and she had her ten- and twelve-year-old daughters with her. We're talking in the office and this woman looks to be about thirty-five.

"I went out of the office and said to one of the guys, 'I think its one of the middle ones, go clean him off.' You know, they foam. The guy ran out to clean them up and then came in and nodded his head that they had them all set.

"I'm going to show her the older guy first. Then she will know what a dead man looks like now. I undid the blanket.

"'Oh, Henry!' she bawled out.

"The girls are outside and hear their mommy crying and they start crying. But she handled it real well. I give her a minute or so. I said, 'Ma'am, would you like us to leave? I'll be just outside the door.'

"She said, 'No.' She stood up and wiped the tears from her eyes. We stepped outside the door.

"She said, 'You know, I don't know what to do. I've lost everything, everything.' Then she turns to me and puts a hand on my shoulder and says, 'I feel sorry for you.'

"Of course, my crew is standing around and everyone has a lump in their throat. The little girls are crying and holding onto mommy.

"'Ma'am I don't understand. You feel sorry for me?'

"'Yes. I only have to go through this once, you must have to go through this every week.'

"My God, that stuck in my throat! I never forgot that."

McAdams next assignment took him to isolated duty in Japan, and when he returned, he received command of Station Umpqua River, Oregon. He then received a year's duty testing the then-new 41-foot utility boats at various locations on the East Coast. By now McAdams was a master chief petty officer. His next assignment was in command of the motor lifeboat school at Cape Disappointment for two years; he left because of a "difference of opinion" with the commanding officer of Station Cape Disappointment. McAdams returned to Station Yaquina Bay, this time as officer in charge.

McAdams recalled that one of the reasons he retired "began when they wanted to know how many hours you were spending working. When I told them, they said, 'You can't spend that many hours at work.'

"'Well, yes, I can. If you add up total hours on duty.'

"'That's absurd, you can't spend that many hours on duty.' To run that station for that many hours we have to go from twenty men to fifty men and that's why you got forty or fifty men at the stations.

"Then they knocked off the salmon season. Then they cut down on this and that, so your private small boats plummeted, as far as ocean-going. At [Cape Disappointment], you went from seven thousand boats out on a single day. Here at Yaquina Bay in the last few years there'd be one to two thousand boats screaming out into the waves to go salmon fishing and all the commercial boats rushing out to sea. You don't have that now. So the calls plummeted on down and now you are left with forty or fifty men and women.

"Another problem I found just before I got out. Every six months they would send an officer down from the district and that officer would take the crew for half a day. He would tell those people all their rights. He would tell them that the chief cannot do this. If that chief does this, you have the right to do this. That chief does not have the right to do this, that chief cannot do this. I listened to several of these talks and not one time did I ever hear that officer say that you have a responsibility. They always said you have rights and don't let these people get away with anything.

"You have a right to captain's mast. I could hold captain's mast. At captain's mast you are God, jury and the whole shootin' match. You know your people. So most of the time I would say, 'Okay, you got fourteen days restriction on your own. You take it, you do it and there's no bookwork. You're saving money, a whole bunch of paperwork and you are saving any type of documentation.' This was great and that was it. They knew that. Then all of a sudden, these officers come along and say, you got rights, take a summary courts-martial. Now the guy says I don't want a captain's mast, I'll get fourteen days. I want a summary. You couldn't restrict them if they were up for a summary, because that's giving them punishment before the trial. So the guy's off. Hell, he's doin' the same thing again, he don't give a shit. You lost your authority, so the guys didn't give a shit about your authority. Why should I do what he says because I can do this, this and this. The officer can get me off and the chief is going to foul up the paperwork anyways. I got my rights and I got an officer backing me up. Pretty soon you lost him. Then what did you lose? You started to lose your training. The guy says, 'I don't have to know this, why should I?' You lose this down the line. If you don't have authority, you have chaos and that's happened a lot. Not just the Coast Guard, all the services, the police, everything. There's no respect anymore for the basics. I finally decided to retire. I went out on 1 July 1977.

"Small boat stations do not get the credit they deserve. Most of the officers did not know what went on at the stations, although a few in headquarters and the district did. Most of the warrants in those days—Fancy Pants was the exception—were old lifeboatmen, they'd been around since the Life-Saving Service days. When the Coast Guard took over, the officers wanted nothing to do with these small boat stations. I mean in the old 36-foot lifeboats you were standing on grates, your feet were under water. The boats were heavy, ten and a half tons, you were out in the open. We didn't have the foul weather gear they have now. We had the worse kind of clothes you could have: denim, the worse thing you could have. Nobody heard of hypothermia. You were cold. I had crews laying down on the deck. Eighty-five percent of my people got seasick. That meant my two crewmembers were seasick, so you had double duty. Even if you gave up the wheel, you had to be there to watch. There was no place to huddle. If you went into the engine room, there was just enough room to get in there. It was warm in there, but the diesel fumes, if you weren't sick, you would be. You were cold. You were wet. You were miserable.

"I had people laying in the well deck so seasick and the water going over them. I remember coming back from Siuslaw River one time my crew begged me, 'How long before we get back?' I told them four or five hours. Oh, the spray and green water pouring over the decks. 'Just run us into the surf,' they said. 'I'll give you my car, my next three paychecks. I'll give you my girl friend, I'll give you my wife! You can have anything you want, just run us into the surf and get us off of here.' There are two stages of seasickness: the first is you think you'll die, the second is you're afraid you won't.

"Officers didn't want to do that type of thing. So the enlisted men or the warrant officers would do it. They should just let them do their job.

"Helicopter pilots do a wonderful job, but a helicopter pilot is sitting in a warm seat and he's got it right there. Everything is right there. Like I told them one time, give me a chopper and give me three months and I'll fly a chopper as well as anybody. But they're officers and the jealousy thing comes in.

"With the detailer system they have now, they're plugging holes. They take a guy that's had so much time here and transfer them there without any reference to his experience. If you have a bad head injury you wouldn't go to a foot doctor for help just because he's doctor. No way. Same thing with lifeboat station men that are lifeboatmen. But now there's this mass transfer of people so that no one ever gets it nailed down anymore. I ran [Yaquina Bay] for my last tour. I still have to run the boats to keep my timing. In fact, I have a boat now and I go north each year to Alaska and Canada and spend two months outside Vancouver Island, British Columbia, just cruising. With the sea, you've got to keep your timing sharp. Professional piano players practice constantly. If you don't do this constantly, you don't stay the best. You lose your timing at sea. One thing about being in the service and getting older and doing your job: as long as you have your health, you can keep that timing, keep those other things going. You can be an asset to the situation. But most of the guys as they get older, they get lazy and start running downhill. They start sending the young guys out. Well that's good, the young guys got to get the experience, but the old man has to be there too.

"The spirit of the guys today is still there, just give them a chance. Give them that extra training. I could take a group of people and put them to work and weed out four or five out of, say, the twenty and I would come out with a crew on the other end that would be just so great and they would respect you. They would be a working team. I used to have that here."

Master Chief Boatswain's Mate Thomas D. McAdams, U.S. Coast Guard (Ret.) is still very fit. He is an officer in the local volunteer fire department and is justifiably proud of his more than fifty years of service in rescuing people.

Master Chief McAdams also still has what the military likes to call a command presence. When he fixes his eyes on you to make a point, he has what is best described as "the Master Chief stare." Any veteran will understand that stare. The only concession to age: he no longer smokes cigars because he noticed "a cough." McAdams, more than twenty-six years after retirement, still is capable of running to Station Yaquina Bay's motor lifeboat, donning his modified aviator's helmet, sticking a cigar in his mouth, pushing the throttles forward, and successfully saving someone on the bar.

SCOTTY

Chief Warrant Officer F. Scott "Scotty" Clendenin, U.S. Coast Guard, retired from the service on 5 August 2000, one day after the service's birthday. Clendenin personified the spirit of the U.S. Coast Guard's motor lifeboat stations. He served three times at Station Yaquina Bay and, like McAdams, ended his career as the commanding officer of the unit.[3]

Clendenin graduated high school in Ravenswood, West Virginia, in 1974 then attended two years of college at Glenville State College in Glenville, West Virginia. Clendenin entered the U.S. Coast Guard on 12 July 1976. As a young boy in West Virginia, he recalled that he lay in bed dreaming about saving people. Unlike many others, Clendenin lived out his boyhood dreams. One salty lifeboatman once remarked about Clendenin's many awards for valor, "All Scotty has to do is walk outside, and a medal will fall from the sky and hit him on the head."

Clendenin's fierce dedication to SAR was legendary throughout the stations. A crewman at Yaquina Bay said, "I will call

Mr. Clendenin in the middle of the night about a case and he answers on the first ring, is wide awake and seems to know all about the case. I don't know when he sleeps." Rumor had it that he slept with a scanner next to his bed. An eighteen-year-old at Yaquina Bay said she had been out many hours on a case in high seas and her head was starting to nod when "Mr. Clendenin said something like, 'You can't be tired,' and made a few jokes. I remember thinking, 'This guy has got to be more than twice as old as I am and he doesn't seem the least bit tired.' Then I remembered always seeing him late at night working out on the Stairmaster."

At times there is a strained relationship between commercial fishing people and the crews who may have to rescue them. Clendenin showed a particular concern and sympathy for those who follow the dangerous profession of commercial fishing, and in talks to his crew, he stressed that fishermen were like U.S. Coast Guard people—both made a living in a very dangerous environment.

Clendenin's abilities and reputation in high surf came to the fore during the *Rain Song* rescue on Thursday, 15 April 1993, at Yaquina Bay. At the time Clendenin was a chief petty officer and executive petty officer (XPO) of the station.

During the afternoon of the fifteenth, the 42-foot charter fishing vessel *Rain Song* interrupted its charter due to rain squalls and low visibility. The vessel's captain faced an uneasy sight as he approached the bar: breakers of at least sixteen to twenty feet. This meant a rough passage for the passengers, but the charter vessel could handle the crossing. As so often happens in heavy breakers, without warning, a "tremendous breaker" hit the vessel and the boat capsized. Twenty-two people now struggled in dangerously high breakers. With the sea water temperature at forty-six degrees Fahrenheit, hypothermia added to the deadly situation.

When *Rain Song* went over, sea water activated the EPIRB. A U.S. Coast Guard aircraft on patrol received the beacon's signal and relayed the information to Station Yaquina Bay and a helicopter unit at Newport. Chief Clendenin immediately got underway in a 30-foot surf rescue boat, CG-30618, with his crewman Machinery Technician 3d Class Jon P. Busier. Scott's boat, the fastest, led the station's two 44-foot motor lifeboats into the surf. Once near the reported area of capsizing, Chief Clendenin assigned the motor lifeboats to two different search patterns while he maneuvered through seas almost as high as his boat was long.

In the rain, blowing spray and plunging surf, Clendenin spotted five desperate survivors clinging to a life ring. Two had serious hip injuries and all were hypothermic and barely managing to hold onto the flotation device. Clendenin acted quickly. He began to maneuver his single-screw craft toward the people in the water. Later, even in the official report, the skill needed even to approach the survivors comes through. "The slightest mistake in maneuvering," reads the report, "could have caused the boat to crash down onto the victims."

Words can not do justice to the scene, but somehow, in the rain and plunging seas, Chief Clendenin brought the 30-footer alongside the helpless survivors. Two of the victims weighed over 250 pounds each. As the last survivor came aboard, the SRB took a large breaking wave, slamming Chief Clendenin, Busier, and the last two survivors to the deck.

Clendenin knew the seas were too rough for a helicopter hoist, so he now set about getting survivors to shore. As he faced the tempest of the bar, a series of large waves bore down upon the 30-footer. To keep from broaching, Clendenin turned into the breakers. Once clear, the surfman again maneuvered to cross. Another series of sixteen- to twenty-two-foot waves plunged toward the craft, and again the surfman put the bow into the seas. He turned the SRB for a third attempt at crossing the bar, and "several 22-foot breakers [came] over the top of his 30-foot rescue craft." Yet Clendenin continued on, and he made it.

An awaiting ambulance took the survivors to a hospital. In the meantime, one of the 44-foot motor lifeboats lost its steering. The other motor lifeboat took the disabled craft into tow and started toward the bar. Without hesitation, Clendenin again set out in the 30-footer toward the bar. He crossed the bar and met up with the two motor lifeboats. Chief Clendenin escorted the boats and used the radio to call out the location of large waves to the other coxswains.

For his work on this dangerous April afternoon, Chief F. Scott Clendenin earned the Coast Guard Medal. What happened later at the awards ceremony would have audiences in disbelief if it were presented on the silver screen. Rear Adm. John W. Lockwood, commander of the Thirteenth U.S. Coast Guard District, the mayor of Newport, and Capt. Michael McCormack, Chief Clendenin's group commander, assembled at the station and were about to present the award when the wail of the SAR alarm sounded. The first boat crew ran to the motor lifeboat. Witnesses later reported they thought Admiral Lockwood was going to have to tackle Chief Clendenin to keep him from running to the surf rescue boat instead of completing the awards presentation.

A senior chief once related that if you were from another station and you brought your boat into Clendenin's station, his crew was waiting with buckets of soapy water to help scrub down your boat and the cook was in the galley making hot food for you. His station was always immaculate and its boats literally shone.

In recent years, the leadership of the service seems anxious to make sure people know how to handle stress. Clendenin had his own unique way. One old salt recalled what happened at a conference on stress called by Clendenin's group commander. The commander asked each of his commanding officers what they did to handle stress. One said that he took walks on the beach with his wife, and others had similar responses. Then came Clendenin's turn. "I fight fires," he told the group commander. On his off-duty time, Clendenin worked as a volunteer fire fighter.

Although he received the Coast Guard Medal, Clendenin once recalled that the case he is most proud of is the saving of a small child earlier in his career at Station Tillamook Bay, Oregon, in 1986. On Sunday morning, 5 October 1986, during heavy fog and strong winds, Station Tillamook Bay's communications watch-stander responded to a call on the CB about a small motorboat caught in the beach breakers and receiving hard blows by the waves. The ready crew started the 30-foot SRB and the 44-foot motor lifeboat. Before the crew departed, the CB's speaker in the station's communication room crackled with "They just capsized, and there's three people hanging onto the side of the boat."

Clendenin, then a boatswain's mate first class and operations petty officer of the station, and Machinery Technician 1st Class Glenn Trapp, called into the station that they were on the way. No sooner had Trapp walked into the operations room than the CB brought more information. The people clinging to the boat had drifted close enough to the beach to wade ashore. One person, however, was missing: a six-year-old boy, Ezequiel Estrella. Clendenin, Machinery Technician 3d Class William Benecke, and Machinery Technician 3d Class Rick Darr drove to the location in the station's four-by-four beach rig. They continued receiving information on the boat via radio.

While the motor lifeboat, SRB, and a helicopter searched, Clendenin, Benecke and Darr picked up the survivors who had made it to the beach. Clendenin spotted the overturned boat about twenty-five feet from the beach. Wearing his survival gear, he plunged into the heavy surf and swam to the boat. "Seeing no debris, I climbed on top of the boat and began to pound on it with my survival knife," Clendenin said. "It was hard to hear with the roar of the breakers."

On the beach, Machinery Technician 3d Class Todd Quinton, who had followed the beach rig, reeled out the cable on the beach rig's winch and attached it to the bow of the capsized boat. Twenty minutes had elapsed since the first CB call. Hearing no sounds from within the boat, Clendenin slid off it and prepared to make his way shoreward when he noticed "a small hand sticking out from beneath the boat." Breakers continued pounding the boat and Clendenin could not free the child.

Clendenin called for the eighteen bystanders on the beach to help lift the thirty-eight-hundred-pound boat high enough for him to pull the child from underneath before the breaking waves brought the boat down upon the child. Among those straining to lift the boat was the commanding officer of Tillamook Bay, Chief Warrant Officer Robert Steiner, dressed in a three-piece suit he had been wearing in church when he responded to the call. "The boy's been found! The boy's been found!" Clendenin broadcast on the CB. The work of everyone on the beach successfully rescued Ezequiel Estrella.

On 5 August 2000, Chief Warrant Officer F. Scott Clendenin retired from the U.S. Coast Guard, his last command having been the commanding officer of Yaquina Bay. Retirement did not mean Clendenin walked away from search and rescue, however. He remained on the Newport Volunteer Fire Department, and almost three years after his retirement, on 6 June 2003, Clendenin again worked SAR in the Pacific Ocean. Just north of the Yaquina Bay Station, at Nye Beach, two young girls, eight and ten years old, became trapped in a strong rip tide. Two bystanders, a father and son, entered the dangerous surf to help the girls. The rip tide then trapped the would-be rescuers.

Station Yaquina Bay sent two 47-foot motor lifeboats to the scene, while a U.S. Coast Guard helicopter from the Air Facility at Newport also departed, but without a rescue swimmer. Newport's volunteer fire department and an ambulance also received the call.

Clendenin was the fire department's rescue swimmer. He entered the surf and helped the father to the beach. Just at this time, the 47-foot motor lifeboat arrived in the area and began pulling out the two girls. The twenty-one-year-old son of the rescued man went under; spotters on the beach could not locate him.

The helicopter started to search the area and spotted the young man below the surface of the water. Clendenin, knowing the helicopter did not have a rescue swimmer, entered the surf. He, too, shortly found himself "caught in the surf." The helicopter crew spotted Clendenin struggling and dropped the rescue basket near him. Clendenin managed to swim to the basket. Once Clendenin was in the basket, the crewman on board the helicopter hoisted him to safety and the helicopter continued the search.

The rescue helicopter again located the young man and Clendenin was lowered into the sea. He began a search in the water and "located the man about five feet below the water." Clendenin later wrote that he "dove down and after several attempts . . . was able to pull the man to the surface and swim him to the [rescue] basket." The helicopter immediately brought the man to the beach and fire and ambulance people rushed him to the hospital. Unfortunately, he did not survive. The helicopter returned to pick up Clendenin. He had spent "a total of 32 minutes in the surf."[4]

PART IV
1996–2003

13 | Into the Twenty-first Century

In 1997, the last of the twentieth century's innovations in coastal motor lifeboats entered the U.S. Coast Guard. Formerly the service had designed and built their heavy weather boats at the U.S. Coast Guard Yard, Curtis Bay, Maryland. Breaking with tradition, Textron Marine and Land of New Orleans, Louisiana, designed and built the new 47-footer. Its hull, of marine-grade aluminum, is not the traditional white but gray, with a red slash and "U.S. Coast Guard" in black at the bows. As with its predecessors, the 47-footer can right itself from a rollover. Specifications for the boat require a recovery time of ten seconds. Like other motor lifeboats, it is self-bailing. Powered by two 435-horsepower Detroit Diesel engines, the boat's maximum speed is twenty-five knots, and it is capable of a cruising speed of twenty-two knots. It can operate in sixty knots of wind and twenty-foot breaking surf. Its open bridge is fourteen feet above the water (at the height of the coxswain's eye). Another steering location is from a lower enclosed bridge. Usually, in high surf coxswains and surfmen prefer to use the open bridge. The boat carries a large amount of electronics. Crew size is four. Because the boat's main deck sits high in the water, there is an area, called the "recess" by boatcrews, where rescuers can pull survivors from the water. The 47-foot motor lifeboat is now the service's heavy weather craft. Continuing into the twenty-first century at small boat rescue stations was the 41-foot utility boat and rigid hulled boats of various sizes. Four 52-foot metal motor lifeboats remain in the Pacific Northwest.[1]

I CAME UP AND SAW SOMEONE SWIMMING OUT TO ME

U.S. Coast Guard personnel are lifesavers even off duty. Early on the Sunday afternoon of 26 November 1995, eleven-year-old Clyde J. "C. J." Hubbs, from Chinook, Washington, his thirteen-year-old brother Ed, and three neighborhood young women were looking for something to do. They decided to play under the Astoria-Megler Bridge, the long span that crosses the Columbia River from Washington state to Astoria, Oregon. The boys remembered they had a rope used to secure some belongings to a concrete bridge support pier located out in the river. C. J. and Ed left the young women on the river bank while they raced under the bridge. They ran out over the water along a narrow steel girder that led to the pier. "We were showing off for the girls," Ed remembered. They had been over this girder before. Then C. J. slipped and plunged fifteen feet into the water.[2]

"I know how to swim real good. I'm not scared of the water," C. J. later told interviewers. "But I had on a heavy sweatshirt taking me down. I kept going down and bobbing up. I thought, 'I know I'm not going to get out of this.'"

"I saw him hit the water," Ed said, "and ran to get the rope. But I couldn't get the knot untied. Then he was too far out. I yelled to the girls to flag down cars and get Dad." Ed ran back to the shoreline and began running along the bank helplessly and yelling after his brother.

The Columbia River that the eleven-year-old plunged into was under the influence of the incoming tide, causing a swift current to sweep C. J. upstream. Washington State Patrol officers later reported "currents in this particular area are amongst some of the strongest on the entire river. There are often large whirlpools just off the rocky riverbank." The river temperature did not top fifty-one degrees.

The young women had managed to stop motorists. More than fifty people stood by the river trying to figure out what to do as C. J. bobbed up and down in the rapid current. At just this time, Subsistence Specialist 3d Class Michael E. Early, off duty as a cook from Cape Disappointment Station, approached the bridge on his way to Portland, Oregon, with a friend and her son. Early thought there must be a wreck and decided to stop to see if he could help. Once out of his car, he heard children yelling that their friend was in the water. He turned, and there, at least seventy-five yards off-shore, bobbed C. J. Early yelled for someone to call the U.S. Coast Guard and the sheriff's department as he ran to the shoreline.

Early threw off his coat and ran upriver, trying to judge where he could best intercept the floundering boy. Just before entering the water, someone tied a rope to Early's waist. He plunged into the numbing water. "I was scared beyond all belief," he later admitted. During the four minutes of grueling swimming, Early continually called out to C. J., attempting to reassure him and trying to get him to swim toward his rescuer.

Ten minutes had passed since C. J. had plunged into the cold water. The boy had gone under a number of times. "You think that when you drown that it's going to hurt and you'll freak out," said C. J. later. "It wasn't like that. It was like being in a nice, comfortable bed, looking around where it's all quiet. As I bobbed up and down, I saw bubbles coming out of my mouth each time I went under and started seeing stars with red. It was real quiet. Then I came up again and saw someone swimming out to me."

As Early approached C. J., he felt "the lifeline to which he was secured dragging him under, yet he feared to untie it because he was unsure he would be able to make it ashore on his own." Early kept the thrashing boy at arm's length while trying to calm him down and prevent him from climbing on top of him. Once

Early had C. J. securely in his grasp, onlookers ashore pulled them to safety.

The Washington State Patrol and an aid car arrived and quickly transported C. J. to the hospital for treatment of hypothermia. Trooper Scott Johnson later reported that "undeniably" had Early not acted "without hesitation, and without regard for his personal safety, C. J. would have perished." Trooper Johnson noted, "Early quietly left the scene without taking any credit for his actions." Johnson believed Early "deserve[d] recognition for his heroism."

On 29 July 1996, Rear Adm. J. David Spade, commander, Thirteenth U.S. Coast Guard District awarded Subsistence Specialist 3d Class Michael E. Early the Gold Life Saving Medal, the seventh highest award for heroism in peacetime that an enlisted person at a small boat station can receive. Early also received a letter from Washington state senator Sid Snyder and a Certificate of Commendation from Governor Mike Lowry.

The written report made by Michael E. Early's commanding officer, Lt. Michael White, describes what is best about the crews of the U.S. Coast Guard's small boat stations: "Early's effort was a selfless act that displayed the qualities the community has always valued in our Coast Guard Men and Women: a willingness to act, even at extreme risk, and a sense of duty, particularly when lives are at stake. His dedication, professionalism, and humanitarian service are commendable and represent the fact that on or off-duty, members of our service are Always Ready."

THE CRAZIEST THING I EVER DID

Many people feel the personnel of the Ninth Coast U.S. Guard District, the Great Lakes, go into hibernation during the winter months. The actions of the crew of Station Charlevoix, Michigan, on the night of 10 February 1996 defy this notion.[3]

The day started bright and sunny, but then the skies began to cloud over. A freezing rain began to fall, and by dark an almost blinding snowstorm struck with thirty-mile-an-hour winds—not unusual winter weather for this northern Lake Michigan town.

At approximately 8:05 P.M., the communications watchstander at Station Charlevoix received a call from a nearby resident who claimed there was someone out on the ice screaming for help. Boatswain's Mate 2d Class Jeffery Kihlmire and two other crewmen were on duty at the time. "The watchstander piped [paged] us to go out to the berm, which is right across the street from the station," he recalled. "When we reached the berm, we could hear hollering. We could just barely see something on the ice." Just barely observable in the winter darkness was a snowmobiler in the water.

"Myself and another crewman, Fireman Garret Powell, ran out into the garage and got into our dry suits and we grabbed our shore ice rescue equipment," Kihlmire related. "The watchstander ran back into the comcenter [communications center] and started making phone calls to get more people down to the location and get the fire department. My wife, Pam, was visiting me at the station at the time. She had six years in the Coast Guard before we got married. Even though she was out of the service, her training probably helped when she went in and helped make telephone calls. They called the fire department and the rest of our crew. The call came in at 8:05, and by 8:08 myself and my crewman were on our way out to get to them with our line pack and ice slide."

The snowmobiler struggled approximately two hundred yards offshore, right in an area where the ice is always thin. Earlier, freezing rain had added to the danger. Kihlmire described the ice as "porous, like a sponge," and anywhere "from one-quarter to three inches thick." The rotted ice made it almost impossible for anyone to walk across it.

In this type of case, according to Kihlmire, "you wear a dry suit and a Type 3 lifejacket, which is like a fishing vest and looks almost like a down vest. You also wear wet suit gloves and whoever goes out for the rescue is at the end of a tethered line in a harness. You carry a boat hook to tap the ice. When you get into thin ice you can hear a distinct thud rather than a crisp sound. When you're crawling, the boat hook also helps to distribute your weight so you can go onto thinner ice, while someone without the boat hook would have real trouble crossing. Plus, you can reach out with it if they're conscious."

When Kihlmire and Powell arrived, they saw one person on the ice. They started over the thicker portions of the ice and then reached the area of thin ice. Interestingly, Fireman Powell earlier that morning had just started learning ice rescue; it was the first time he had been on the ice. Now, on his second time on the ice, he found himself in a life-and-death situation. Kihlmire recalled that "going out the visibility was poor, with the snow coming down sideways and dark. So there I was, crawling on my belly across the ice, with a flashlight in my mouth to see where I was going, in the dark and in a snowstorm. Every few feet my elbows would break through the ice as I crawled. I went a good twenty-five yards that way. The man was somewhat conscious when I got to him. First thing I asked him: what happened, was he on a snowmobile? If he had been driving and smashed through the ice, you could be dealing with internal injuries and have to be careful of how you move him around. I also asked him if there was anybody with him. His level of consciousness was so low that he said no.

"I started to work him out. My line tender, Powell, would pull us a little bit and we'd break through. I would get him back up on the ice and we'd break through again. Both my weight and his weight were just too much. After what seemed like forever, but it was only a manner of a few minutes, we got two more of our crew out there on the ice with us. One of the other fellows came out with a sled—a plastic ski tote with flotation tubes on each side—and we got the person in the sled and even that kept breaking through. So, it was real slow, arduous work before we finally got him to thicker ice and finally off the ice. As we timed it later, we actually had him off the ice in about ten, fifteen minutes."

The man was placed in an ambulance and started toward the emergency room. "When they got him in the ambulance and removing all his wet clothes," Kihlmire said, "they tried to get his arms down and he was so froze up they couldn't get his arms down. Of the paramedics that arrived on scene, the one that was cutting off the clothes from his lower extremities later found it was her son-in-law. She didn't recognize him; he was so blue and distorted from being in the cold. His body core temperature when he got to the hospital was eighty-six, I think, so he was very near death."

The story is not yet complete. Once the man started to come to in the hospital, the rescuers learned that the man's brother was on another snowmobile right behind him. "So we turned right around and went right back out again," said Kihlmire. "Half of our station had been recalled. This time we launched the ice skiff and broke ice in there as far as we could, but his brother had gone under the ice sometime before. The nearest they could figure, before we were notified, he was out there for approximately twenty-five minutes to a half-hour. We searched for a long time, and so did other agencies, but his brother has not been found."

Later, rescuers learned the two brothers, each on his own machine, had started across the ice, become disoriented in the weather, and stopped. Once they stopped, their machines broke through the thin ice.

In 1997, at his new station at Cape Disappointment, Washington, Kihlmire, by then a boatswain's mate first class, related, "In eleven years in the Coast Guard, the ice rescue is probably the craziest thing I ever did. When I enlisted in the Coast Guard, it's the last thing I ever thought I would be doing, crawling across the ice on my stomach in a whiteout in the middle of Lake Charlevoix in Michigan. It's something I would do again if I had to, but it's not something I would want to do all the time. Funny part is the flashlight made it back after I got to him. I put it inside the lifejacket. That's one of the things I didn't lose."

For the actions on this cold, stormy February night in Michigan, Jeffery Kihlmire won the Coast Guard Commendation Medal. Garret Powell, the line tender, received the Coast Guard Achievement Medal, and the two sled tenders and another seaman won letters of commendation. Everyone at the station that had something to do with the rescue, including the fire department personnel who reported into the unit to help, received the Team Award. Pam Kihlmire also received the Team Award for working the telephones at the station. "She may now have more medals than me," said Jeffery Kihlmire.

IT'S MY JOB

In the predawn hours of 29 December 1996, Station Grays Harbor, Washington, responded to a call from the 58-foot wooden-hulled crabber *Lee Rose.* Her skipper radioed he was twelve miles northwest of Grays Harbor. *Lee Rose* was battling eight-foot seas and fifty-knot winds along with rain and hail showers. The crabber was taking on water.

Chief Warrant Officer Randy Lewis, the commanding officer, recalled, "It had been stormy the night on the 28th before I went to bed, near ten o'clock. We had about three inches of snow and my kids were going crazy; they were going to have a lot of fun the next day playing in the snow.

"The station called about three in the morning and said they had this guy taking on water, so I drove in and as I got into the station the snow had pretty much changed to rain. I got in and started to figure who, what, and where. There was a helo on the way from Astoria, Oregon, to the south, but they were really fighting the weather. The wind was coming out of the northwest and was really screaming, during the whole case it was probably forty to fifty knots, with gusts upwards to seventy to seventy-five. We decided to go with the *Invincible,* the 52-foot motor lifeboat, and the 44-footer. I would be the coxswain on the *Invincible* and Boatswain's Mate First Class Daniel L. Smock would be the coxswain on the other boat. We were still on our holiday routine and working with fewer people in the duty sections, so the 44-footer had a crew of three and I had four."[4]

Lee Rose shaped a course toward Grays Harbor bar. The fishing vessel *Jamie Marie* escorted the crabber until they rendezvoused with the two U.S. Coast Guard boats two to three miles north of the entrance. Smock recalled, "It was a pretty decent ride out with about three to four feet of wind chop coming out of the east. About fifteen minutes after we got on scene, the temperature went from about thirty degrees, with a thirty-knot east wind, to fifty-five degrees, and about a forty-knot southwest wind. Even the weather buoy reports changed. The seas went from a three- to four-foot chop to a southwest fourteen- to twenty-foot swell at about a five-second interval. It was close, choppy and blowing hard. The windshield on the 44-footer fogged up and I couldn't see until the windshield warmed enough. The warm front was like a curtain rolling right over us."

"The weather was so bad," said Lewis, "that the helicopter went right over us and couldn't see our lights. We actually got on scene before the helo. They had to almost get right down on the deck before they could see anything. On the way out, I kept look-ing at the range marks for reference. I looked back once and said, 'Crap! The fog's moved in.' One of the crewmen turned around and said, 'No, the lights went out.' The whole town lost power.

"Comms [communications] were bad and we were basically on our own. Group Astoria called the helo and said they had no lights at the airport at all. The helo called me and asked if I wanted him to stay around. I said you're not going to put a rescue swim-mer in this stuff, especially with the boats around, you'd better work your way home. I talked to one of the pilots later and he said they put the helicopter at four hundred feet to miss anything on their route and started toward Astoria along the coast. The weather was so bad they figured they were only making ten to twenty knots speed over the ground."

The four boats started into the shelter of Westport, Washington. *Jamie Marie* went first, followed by the two U.S. Coast Guard boats and *Lee Rose. Lee Rose* "had pumps running and all he could tell us was water was coming into his engine room from somewhere and he was just keeping ahead of it," said Lewis. "As we got nearer the entrance, there's an area called 'The Triangle,' which ends up being an ugly area for waves. The chan-nel heads to the southwest and there's a green line [the line that represents the left-hand side of a channel coming in from the sea] that goes to the north and west and the area between the two ends up ugly. He was going into that area. He started to take some good swells. I had just turned to a crewman and said, 'Man, if he has troubles down here, we're not going to be able to help him.' About five minutes later, he took a series of three about twenty-five-footers that just stood the boat on its stern.

"He called and said his crewman had just come up and said the pumps weren't keeping up and the water was coming in fast. He said he could either run offshore or keep trying to run inshore.

"So I told him you got basically two choices: offshore it's just going to get bigger and it would take at least a half hour's running heading in before you get into good enough water where we can get alongside to pass a pump. His decks were awash and a pump would flood out.

"He said, 'I am going to put a crewman on the wheel and look for myself.' He came back and said, 'Nope, the steering pump is going under at anytime. I am amazed that I still have steering.'

"I really thought it was time for him to get off it. I'd had some of those old, crusty skippers who will start to argue with you. Somehow, someway he was going to do it. But the skipper was a younger guy and he decided to leave the boat. I called the helo and told them they'd better come back and stand by just in case. They turned and, now with the wind on their tail, they came back at a speed later calculated to be over two hundred miles per hour."

Jamie Marie, hearing the radio traffic, and in the best tradition of the sea, turned from seeking safe moorage and returned to the scene to use their strong sodium lights to illuminate the area.

Lewis was now maneuvering a 52-foot motor lifeboat, a craft that is noted for its rolling when rough—one crewman called it like a weeble-wobble toy—keeping track of the 44-foot motor lifeboat, a crabber in serious trouble, and coordinating a helicopter and *Jamie Marie.* All of this is enough to do in a dry office, but imagine it on a windy, wet deck.

Chief Warrant Officer Lewis suggested the fishing crew, now in their exposure suits, jump from the stern one at a time and a motor lifeboat would pick up each person. "I talked it over on the radio with the CO," said Smock, "and decided to take the first pickup. The skipper of the *Lee Rose* would keep steering right into the swells at a slow bell [slow speed] and have a crewman walk to the stern and I'd be sitting right behind him. I'd peel off and pick him up and the 52 was sitting right behind me and he'd pull up into position and then I'd stand off."

"On the first pickup," said Seaman Daniel C. Butenschoen, a crewman on board the 44-foot motor lifeboat, "we were in our surf belts, clipped to the boat, and we worked ourselves down to the well deck, the lowest point in the middle of the boat, where it is easiest to grab a person in the water. I didn't even see him jump off the boat until all of a sudden I see something floating in the water. 'Is that him? Oh, crap!'

"Petty Officer Smock did a great job in getting us alongside the person in the water. For some reason we couldn't get the boat's lifelines unsnapped. Our hands were really cold. We're trying to pick him up with the lifelines in place. I'm trying to bring this guy, who's all crinkled up from the cold, over the lines while Mike's trying to bring him under. So, finally, we just picked him up over the lines, checked him out and got him up to the coxswain's flat and put him into one of the extra surf belts. Then we backed off and let the *Invince* go in to pick up the second person."

"Fortunately, all the people in the water were conscious when we pulled them out, which helps a lot," Lewis said. "It takes a lot of courage on the 52-footer to get someone out of the water in rough seas because of the high freeboard. There's at least one guy who has to belt himself in at the base of the two stanchions of the lifelines, lay on his belly and the other two guys either hold onto his feet or sit on top of them as he reaches out over the side. So you're hanging over the side of the boat and when the boat rolls one way you go down to about your chest in the water and then when you roll the other way, you can easily hear the props breaking suction. The exhaust is right there and you're getting that in the face. Actually, it is probably better to do it at night time, because you can't see the seas coming. In the day time, you look down the hull and see all those breakers coming at you. Makes you want to do it a lot quicker."

"We were clipped into the lifeline, so we could slide up and down the boat," said Machinery Technician Third Class Randy Merritt, a crewman on the 52-footer. "I was clipped on the bottom lifeline. I grabbed him and then the other two crewmen grabbed him. I then clipped onto the top lifeline and helped them bring him on board. Petty Officer Merritt had done this before, but it was the first time for the rest of the crewmen. So it came down to a test. Whether we were going to be able to do what we trained for. Our adrenalin was so honked, we did it so fast, we were all proud of ourselves.

"We asked the *Lee Rose* crewman if he was all right and he said he was fine. We put him in a surfbelt and took him up to where the commanding officer was at on the wheel. The CO then backed out and the 44-footer went in for the third person."

"After the third guy went off," said Lewis, "I talked to the skipper of the *Lee Rose* and asked if he felt safe pulling the boat out of gear so it wouldn't just steam ahead offshore and collide with somebody. He said, 'Yeah, he'd do it.'

"You learn a lot in hindsight. I didn't tell him which way to jump, so he jumped off the down slope quarter of the boat like his crewmen."

"The skipper jumped off the leeward side of the stern and the boat was drifting in on him," said Smock.

"He paddled like mad and was able to get fifty to seventy feet away from the stern," said Lewis.

"There was no room for the 52 to go in and make the pickup. We were just standing by watching," Smock recalled. "Oh, shit! This is gonna get ugly. At just that time there must have been a sixteen- to eighteen-foot break hit the *Lee Rose* broadside and came over the top of the wheel house. All we saw was white water completely over the top of the wheel house, the boat heeled over and then the swell let go of it. The white water that came over the top hit the skipper in the water and washed him about twenty yards away from the boat, which was far enough for the *Invince* to pick him up."

Both Smock and Lewis remarked on how much the sodium lights of the *Jamie Marie* helped in spotting people in the water on this dark, stormy night with crab pots also floating in the area. The 44-foot and 52-foot motor lifeboats then started in over the bar. The sea still had a few punches left, however.

"I let the 44-footer go in first," said Lewis.

"On the transit in," said Smock, "we had the opportunity to surf a nice fourteen-footer. It was just a big, sluffing sea break. I got slapped broadside and we heeled over seventy to eighty degrees. It was an easy transit, except for night time when the wind is blowing, the visibility is low, and there is about sixteen feet of white water. The pucker factor on that one. . . . I know the *Invincible* got slapped hard."

"Coming in," said Lewis, "we were being set toward the north jetty, so we had to run in the trough. At night it's hard getting the proper depth perception. At one point we skirted around a swell and the next thing I saw was a wall of water coming at us. I thought about turning into it, but, nope, I wouldn't have time. So, I yelled for everyone to hold on. We rolled far enough to dump fuel out of the vents. I wouldn't want to do that in a 44-footer."

"A wall of water hit us on the way in," related Boatswain's Mate Third Class Brian Gaunt. "If I wasn't clipped in, I'd probably gone over the side. Took a couple more swells and drank about two hundred gallons of water. Pretty scary ride, not being able to see the waves at night. That's when you get scared. People who say they aren't scared, there's something wrong with them. It's all right to be scared. At the time you're doing it you're not scared." However, one crewman later said, "Uh, uh, at the time *I was scared!*"

The two motor lifeboats with the four rescued fishermen finally made the safety of the harbor. *Lee Rose* eventually drifted at least twenty miles, to Point Grenville, before breaking up.

For their work in the early morning hours of 29 December 1996, Randy D. Lewis and Daniel L. Smock received the Coast

Guard Commendation Medal. Crewmen George L. Paradis, Daniel C. Butenschoen, Mike Fratusco, Randy Merritt, and Brian Gaunt all received Coast Guard Achievement Medals.

Later, when asked if he would do it again, Boatswain's Mate 3d Class Brian Gaunt replied, "Yeah. It's my job."

NOT ON MY WATCH

Michael Carola of Oakland, Maryland, did not have the money for college, and, in fact, college did not interest him. After graduating high school in 1998, Carola, who was not sure what else to do, enlisted in the U.S. Coast Guard. He felt the service "seemed the most exciting."[5] Carola enlisted under a guaranteed district option. After finishing boot camp, and using his guaranteed district option, Carola requested duty in the Thirteenth U.S. Coast Guard District, which includes Washington and Oregon. He wanted to serve in Oregon. Most veterans will quickly recognize what happened to his guaranteed option. On 17 November 1998, Carola reported to Station Oregon Inlet, on North Carolina's Outer Banks. Someone in personnel apparently thought Oregon Inlet was in the state of Oregon. Carola "did not complain a lot," as his family had vacationed on the Outer Banks and he enjoyed the area.

Carola did not know what career pattern to follow in the U.S. Coast Guard. Boatswain's Mate 2d Class Wally Cutchin, in his section, became Carola's mentor. "I saw what he did and it made me want to be a Boatswain's Mate. He was an awesome boat driver and was always there for new guys who had questions and problems. His crew looked up to him."

On Saturday, 6 May 2000, just before his alarm clock went off, Michael Carola, now a seaman, heard Boatswain's Mate 2d Class David Burns running down the hall of the barracks pounding on the doors of the first boat crew. Burns yelled, "We got a boat that hit the bridge!" Carola joined Burns, Machinery Technician 3d Class Francisco Romero, Boatswain's Mate 3d Class Scott O'Brien, and Seaman Amie Boyd on board the 47-foot motor lifeboat CG-47201. The crew threw off the mooring lines, and the motor lifeboat started toward the Bonner Bridge. Carola later recalled that the coxswain, Burns, maneuvered the boat through an unmarked channel "used by experienced coxswains during good water. The locals call it the cut-through." It cut the passage from "about ten minutes at 1.5 nautical miles, versus twenty minutes and 4.5 to 5 nautical miles through the regular channel." Over the radio, the motor lifeboat crew learned that a 50-foot sport fishing vessel, *Little Fly Fisherman,* had struck the bridge and was going down with five people on board. Carola later said that the crew could hear the group talking with the fishing vessel over the radio for five minutes and then communications with the vessel were lost.

It took Oregon Inlet Station's motor lifeboat ten minutes to reach the Bonner Bridge. The bridge has two U-shaped fender systems to protect the concrete pilings. "As we came around from the west side," said Carola, the motor lifeboat crew spotted *Little Fly Fisherman* submerged. "We saw a bunch of people hanging onto the outriggers [of the fishing vessel]. The bow was down. This was pretty intense for six in the morning." The motor lifeboat crew now realized they had seven people in the water. "Seven faces were staring at us, like, 'Thank goodness, here's the Coast Guard!'"

The location of the submerged fishing vessel made the motor lifeboat crew work within a very confined space with a strong four-knot current. Burns, the coxswain, decided to work the motor lifeboat as close as possible to the survivors hanging onto *Little Fly Fisherman*'s outriggers. Burns wanted his crew to determine if anyone needed immediate help. Once he maneuvered into position, the people in the water said there was an elderly man, Douglas Eaker, who had hip problems and could not swim well. "We put our main focus on him," said Carola.

O'Brien threw a life ring with a line attached to Eaker. "Because of the four-knot current," he recalled, "I actually had to hit the people with the life ring to get it to them."[6] Eaker put his arms and head through the life ring and let go of the outrigger. Carola recalled that the rescue crew expected "just [to pull Eaker] over to the boat. . . . [I received] the worse rope burn I've ever got.

The current grabbed [Eaker]. He went about three to five feet in five seconds. . . . I remember [O'Brien] let go of the line. His hand was just smokin'." Eaker ended against the fender system of the bridge.

Another person clinging to the outrigger of *Little Fly Fisherman* cast off in an attempt to help Eaker. Three years after the event, Carola still vividly remembered the next few seconds. The man "went about three feet and just disappeared. Boom! The current sucked him under. [Our crew] started screaming, 'Has anyone got a visual?'" The man "got sucked under the north-side center span and went all the way underwater underneath the channel and got spit out at least six to seven hundred feet from our position." When the man surfaced, so did his hat. "He yelled, 'I got my hat!'"

Another man clutching the fishing vessel's outrigger also tried to reach Eaker. The current set him against a piling covered with sharp barnacles. "To make matters worse," a large cooler from *Little Fly Fisherman* broke loose and the current carried it to Eaker's position. The cooler began battering the elderly Eaker.

The crew increasingly became concerned as Eaker's chin began drooping into the water. Burns tried to maneuver the motor lifeboat closer to him, but the current pushed the bow away. Burns also worried about the current pushing his boat onto the people in the water. And he faced the risk of picking up debris in the propellers. The coxswain decided on a different tactic. He placed the lifeboat's starboard beam against a piling.

O'Brien and Carola leaped onto the piling. O'Brien took a two-inch line with a carabiner, a device used in rock climbing, with him. Both scrambled atop the I-beam pilings to Eaker's location. Carola climbed down the I-beam to water level. O'Brien passed the line to Carola, who wrapped the line around the cooler. O'Brien pulled the cooler up and out of the way.

Eaker understandably began to panic and choke. "I'm trying to calm him down," recalled Carola. "I was trying to grab his wrist. There was an I-beam that was . . . [at] water level and it had a little back spacing to it. I was hoping to pull him up so that he could rest his upper body out of the water. I'm, like, laying horizontally at water level on the I-beam trying to calm the guy and pull him up."

At just about this time, *Little Fly Fisherman* shifted. Another man drifted over to Eaker's and Carola's position. "So it was the two guys besides me. I was in the middle. The other guy was sliced up. I asked how he was doing. He said, 'I'm doing great. We just got to get my father out of here.' There are now two sons who are now looking at us to do something."

O'Brien and Carola knew they had to think of a solution. The current was too strong for Carola to swim Eaker to the motor lifeboat. Further, the same current prevented the coxswain from maneuvering too close to the position. "I looked down at [Eaker]. I realized he wasn't saying anything. I started shaking him, asking if he was okay. He looked up at me and said, 'Let me go, I'm going to die.'[7] Then he blacked out. His head fell back. I said, 'No, you're not. Not today. Not on my watch.'"[8] Carola dropped into the water in front of Eaker to block the force of the current and reposition him in the life ring.

Three years after the event, Carola recalled that "all of a sudden I got this weird idea. The rescue swimmer on a helo has a cable and the helo kind of drags him. Maybe they could do that with the boat. I relayed up to O'Brien what I wanted to do."

Carola yelled to Romero to throw a two-inch line to him. "I wrapped the line around me. I locked onto [Eaker]. I told Romero to make the line off on the forward post and have [Burns] back down hard. I figured if I could hold on for at least five to ten seconds, I would be ripped away from the fender system and [the strong current]." It worked.

Out of the current, Carola swam Eaker over to the motor lifeboat. While trying to get him on board, the crew discovered Eaker's large size. "It took everything we had to get him on board. We started to treat him for hypothermia, he was really blue."

Burns then maneuvered the boat to return to the dock so Eaker could receive immediate medical attention. A line, however, fouled one of the propellers. Fortunately, at just about this time, a charter vessel came alongside and a passenger yelled out that he was a doctor. The motor lifeboat crew transferred Eaker and Boyd to the vessel, and Dr. Jerry Lucas began work on Eaker. The charter vessel returned to its moorings, where emergency medical personnel waited.[9]

Meanwhile, other fishing vessels had arrived on scene and began recovering people from the water. Some, recognizing Carola's technique, tied flotation devices to a line, threw them to the survivors, and pulled them to the boats.

The motor lifeboat returned to bridge area, and Carola and O'Brien helped the two men hanging onto the pilings to the boat. Next they made their way back to the station at five knots, due to the lost propeller. Carola recalled, "That was probably the most sobering time I've [had] on a boat. We were just standing there thinking, Wow! This is what we all wanted to do. We joined for certain reasons, but it's always to be a lifesaver or rescuer. I don't think anyone said a word for the hour it took us to get to the station."

When the boat returned to the station haul out, the officer in charge and executive petty officer met them. "Master Chief Griffith was a guy of few words," Carola remembered, "but he came up to us and said, 'I'm proud of you guys.' He said he wasn't mad about the boat and did not question anything we did. That made us all feel great."

For his heroic actions, Seaman Michael Carola received the Coast Guard Medal and the Association for Rescue at Sea's Gold Medal. Three years later, in an understatement, Michael Carola, now a boatswain's mate third class and serving at Station Yaquina Bay, Oregon, said, "It was a wild day."

THE *MISS BRITTANY* CASE

Beth E. Rasmussen enlisted in the U.S. Coast Guard on 11 September 1997 at the age of nineteen. Her father was a career U.S. Air Force officer, and "after moving every two to three years, my father retired when I was a sophomore in high school and we moved from Springfield, Virginia, to Spokane, Washington, [so that] I would be able to finish high school in the same place I called home." She graduated high school and attended Spokane Falls Community College, mostly "to play basketball and softball."[10]

When asked why she chose to join the U.S. Coast Guard, Beth replied, "My family has a summer cabin on Lake Coeur d'Alene, Idaho. I spent every summer there and learned driving boats and other fun water activities. Being on the water is something I love. It is now even better; I can save lives."

After leaving boot camp, her first assignment was the 378-foot cutter *Mellon* (WHEC-717), home ported in Seattle, Washington. While serving in *Mellon,* she advanced from seaman apprentice, to seaman, and then to boatswain's mate third class. Rasmussen's next assignment, in October 1999, was across country to Station Woods Hole, on Cape Cod, Massachusetts. At that unit, she qualified as a coxswain on the 41-foot utility boat.

The pinnacle of the small boat rescue profession is the surfman level. If you visit with people at the stations, you quickly learn that those who want to qualify for this level try for an assignment to Station Cape Disappointment, Washington, the guardians of the Graveyard of the Pacific. Rasmussen was willing to "mutual," or swap duty stations, in August 2000, which allowed her to serve at this unit noted for its consistently high surf. (The service allows enlisted people with the same qualifications to mutual if their commanding officers approve and the person pays his or her own way.) Rasmussen advanced to boatswain's mate second class in May 2001 and qualified as a coxswain in the 47-foot motor lifeboat. In 2002, she qualified as surfman.

Recent newspaper articles that have decried the state of the U.S. Coast Guard claim that people who serve at the rescue stations can work a staggering eighty-nine hours a week. Despite protestations to the contrary from headquarters, this estimate is too low. Yet some people who serve at the stations, despite these long hours, work additional hours to help others. Rasmussen, for example, after attending the service's Emergency Medical Technician (EMT) School, joined the Pacific County, Washington, Fire Department "to keep [up] my skills." She learned of the formation of a beach rescue team and decided that was what she wanted to do. Rasmussen had to pass a swimming pool test of a timed five-hundred-meter swim, followed by other timed events. Outdoor testing required her to swim fifteen minutes in the breaking surf zone, then swim past the breaking waves. After swimming past the surf zone, she had to swim five hundred meters along the shoreline. The last part of the test required her to pick up a simulated victim offshore and swim back to the beach. Rasmussen also broke in on the rescue jet ski after getting rescue swimmer qualified. She explained that a person needed fifty hours in the beach surf zone, "with numerous simulated rescues, rollovers with recovery of the [jet ski] and personnel rescues. This all took a couple of weeks, but once done, I started doing beach patrol *on my off weekends*" (emphasis added).

On the early morning of 7 August 2001, the communications watchstander at Cape Disappointment received a call from a woman on a cell telephone reporting an overturned boat in the surf in the deadly Peacock Spit area; shortly thereafter, the U.S. Coast Guard received a "hit" from an Emergency Position Indicator Radio Beacon (EPIRB). Lt. Richard J. Burke Jr., the prospective new commanding officer of the Cape Disappointment Station, and Lt. Cdr. Daniel C. Johnson, the commanding officer, hurried to the station's lookout tower to make sure it was not a boat from a previous case.

What the two officers observed was the 45-foot crabber *Miss Brittany*, with three people on board, capsized in the surf. The wind at the time was southwesterly at ten to fifteen miles per hour, with seas four to six feet and swells eight to twelve feet. The executive petty officer of Cape Disappointment, Senior Chief Boatswain's Mate Thomas Karcewski, headed toward the isolated beach on his motorcycle, while other station members followed shortly after that in the station's two beach rigs. The 47-foot motor lifeboat on bar patrol diverted to the area and the station's safe boat got underway. Air Station Astoria dispatched a helicopter to the scene.

Later, Robert Greenfield, the owner and operator of *Miss Brittany*, would tell the U.S. Coast Guard that he had "come around the North Jetty, talked with some fishermen," and it looked like "a nice day." Greenfield ran about twenty crab pots, then happened to look back and saw "a breaker coming in. It curled in my boat and broke my pilothouse windows out. I was pinned in my boat [and] couldn't see anything. I swam to the front of the boat and [found] a little space to breathe and I swallowed a lot of water. The sink drain was giving me an air pocket and I smacked out a piece of plastic, [which] probably saved my life. After about one-half hour, I felt the survival suits [float against me]. I was getting hypothermic, so I put one on. After [*Miss Brittany* drifted into the shallow water near the] beach, I was concerned about the boat settling in the sand and me losing what air I had left. I then heard somebody pounding on the hull, I hit back with some wood that I had found." Greenfield's two crewmen were swept from the boat and lost.

At approximately 7:30 A.M., Rasmussen, at home on her day off, received a message on her pager from the fire department. "The dispatcher noted . . . there were three people in the water off Benson Beach," she recalled. "I immediately threw on my wetsuit and proceeded to the north jetty. When I arrived on scene, about 7:45, the Coast Guard beach rig and another Pacific County Fire Department rescue swimmer, Doug Knutsen, were standing by just up the beach from the overturned vessel, . . . which was one nautical mile northwest of the north jetty. I . . . climbed into the back of Doug's truck with binoculars and began scanning the . . . breakers."

Rasmussen later estimated that the seas were four to six feet and building, with eight- to ten-foot breaking waves five hundred yards offshore. The fire department personnel and U.S. Coast Guard crew swept the area with binoculars and searched the beach area.

Rasmussen would later report that she and Knutsen "decided to walk out to the vessel. *Miss Brittany* was upside down with the stern toward the beach and settling into the sand." Rasmussen remarked that by this time another fire department volunteer had arrived on scene and would be their spotter, watching them carefully as they made their way to the fishing vessel. Rasmussen estimated the vessel lay about two to three hundred yards offshore, with surf in the area of two to four feet. The five-foot ten-inch Rasmussen and Knutsen began their struggle out to the fishing vessel.

"I was abeam of the vessel," Rasmussen recalled, "when Doug Knutsen hopped on the port quarter. I then heard a loud pounding on the hull. Doug . . . hollered, 'Talk to him! . . . I'm going back for a chainsaw!' I climbed onto the hull and started tapping around to find the person's exact location and find . . . the best spot to make a cut. I continued to tap to ensure him I was still there. When Doug returned, he began to cut with the chainsaw, while I continued to hold [onto] his lifejacket. Shortly . . . we had about ten rescuers assisting us."

Once Greenfield was free of the vessel, he informed his rescuers about his two crewmen washed overboard when *Miss Brittany* capsized. Knutsen and Rasmussen continued to tap the rest of the hull just in case the two crewmen had not gone over the side. Once on the beach, Rasmussen continued searching with a Pacific County Fire Department jet ski, towing the fire department's rescue swimmer Greg McLeod on a rescue board behind the ski. They found only debris and the fishing vessel's EPIRB and returned to the beach command post and secured the search.

Later, at 8:30 P.M., Rasmussen, Knutsen, and McLeod arrived back on scene with the intention of making new cuts in the hull to further ensure no one remained trapped within the fish hold. The rescuers found family members had already been at the boat and made a cut but "did not check inside the fish hold due to [the] risk involved. . . . The three of us made our way out to the vessel with our survival gear and flashlights. Doug Knutsen felt out the entire fish hold with negative results. We returned to the beach and secured our search."

In 2001, Boatswain's Mate 2d Class Beth Rasmussen reenlisted for six additional years. "I would love to go to flight school in the future, but not any time soon," she said. "I'm just having too good of a time driving boats, but the Coast Guard will only let me do that for so long before I'll be behind a desk. I want to stay operational throughout my career for as long as I can. Also, my father was a pilot in the Air Force, my uncle was a helo pilot in the Navy and another uncle a pilot for the Air National Guard, so it kinda runs in the family."

Rasmussen married Scott Slade on 26 July 2003. (See below about Scott Slade.) She advanced to boatswain's mate first class on 1 December 2003 and near the end of December found that she and Scott were expecting their first child.[11]

CAPSIZED BOAT IN PEACOCK SPIT

The Labor Day holiday in the United States is traditionally the last of summer vacations. Many Americans who enjoy the water try to cram as much as they can into the long weekend, so the holiday is also the time when rescue stations of the U.S. Coast Guard are particularly active.

On 2 September 2001, Boatswain's Mate 1st Class Christopher D'Amelio, twenty-six, of Cape Disappointment Station, duty rotation meant duty on Labor Day weekend. D'Amelio had entered the U.S. Coast Guard in January 1995. "Tired of college," he decided upon the U.S. Coast Guard because he had spent time "around the ocean . . . surfing."[12] His first duty station was the 378-foot cutter *Sherman* (WHEC-720) at Alameda, California. His next transfer took him to the 110-foot patrol boat *Long Island* (WPB-1342) at Monterey, California. After this, D'Amelio received orders to Cape Disappointment at Ilwaco, Washington, in 1998, which meant a large change from cutters and patrol boats. The lifestyle in coastal Washington state also brought a change: Ilwaco is small and the climate is cool and moist. On Sunday, 2 September, D'Amelio was a surfman with three years of experience at "Cape D."

Across the Columbia River at U.S. Coast Guard Air Station Astoria, Oregon, thirty-seven-year-old Aviation Survival Technician 1st Class Eric T. Forslund also began his duty day. Forslund, from Lakewood, Colorado, had enlisted in the U.S. Coast Guard in April 1988, after serving in the U.S. Marine Corps Reserve. He wanted to change services because the U.S. Coast Guard is always engaged in a mission, such as search and rescue or law enforcement, rather than always training. Forslund, after serving at a number of aviation stations, reported on board Air Station Astoria on 1 August 2001, the same day he advanced to petty officer first class. Sunday, 2 September, was Forslund's second duty day at Astoria. It would prove memorable.[13]

D'Amelio later recalled that, across the river from Astoria, though the day was "nice, we had a huge northwest swell running. The main channel was probably twelve to fourteen feet [in height], sometimes bigger. Clatsop [Spit] was . . . fourteen to sixteen feet, with occasional eighteen feet. Offshore you had that long [Pacific] swell, probably fifteen feet, with a twenty-five-second period. A long, big rolling swell, so when it hits a sandbar, it jacks right up. It was breaking everywhere, but [in] the main channel. Peacock [Spit] was real big."

D'Amelio spent the morning underway on the 47-foot motor lifeboat. "We had something like fifteen cases that day," he recalled. "We had an earlier case of two gentlemen in Peacock Spit that [died.] We could not reach them with the motor lifeboat, but the helo [from Air Station Astoria, across the river] got to them."

Forslund's first case of the day was a hiker who "broke his ankle and couldn't hike out of the cliff he had tumbled down. I was lowered and we executed a routine basket hoist." His next case was being lowered to pick up the bodies of the two men who had drowned in Peacock Spit.

Near noon, D'Amelio and his crew brought their 47-footer into the boat docks to get lunch. The boatswain's mate also wanted to talk with his commanding officer, Lt. Richard J. Burke. Jr. While Burke and D'Amelio talked in the communications room, the motor lifeboat prepared to get underway and stand by at the bar in case of trouble. The coxswain on board the 47-footer was Boatswain's Mate 2d Class Scott E. Slade, who entered the service in September of 1997 from Spokane, Washington. Slade said he "did not know what the Coast Guard was," but on a vacation to Florida he saw a patrol boat and decided to "check out" the service. "I had a couple of years of college, but that wasn't for me."[14] His first unit was at Wrightsville Beach, North Carolina. His next transfer was to Cape Disappointment in 1999.

Another member of the crew, Machinery Technician 3d Class Darrell M. Ryan, was the break-in boat engineer. Ryan, born 9 March 1980 at Clatskanie, Oregon, near Astoria, entered the U.S. Coast Guard on 14 July 1998, because he "grew up on the water and liked being on the water." He thought that the service would be a "good way to make a living, with the bonus of saving lives and helping people."[15]

After boot camp, Ryan attended Machinery Technician School and, upon completing his training, received orders to a station at Carquinez, California. In 2001, Ryan mutualed with another engineer at Cape Disappointment. Ryan wanted to be near his family and his girlfriend.

Just as Petty Officer Slade got underway from the dock, the telephone in the communications room rang. On the line was the duty officer from across the Columbia River at Group Astoria, Oregon, reporting that they had received a cell telephone call from someone on a boat who said "they were between the lighthouses and they were taking breaks and all of a sudden the guy said, 'Oh, shit!' and cut out."[16]

Burke and D'Amelio talked about the situation for "about two seconds," then told the watchstander to sound the SAR alarm. Slade, maneuvering the motor lifeboat out into the river, recalled he "heard the SAR alarm go off and 'capsized boat in Peacock Spit.'" Slade knew there needed a surfman on board, so he returned to the dock to await D'Amelio.

In "about three minutes," D'Amelio was on board and underway. He later recalled that they could not go full speed for the entire two and a quarter miles to the last reported area of the boat. "[We made] fourteen to fifteen knots, [because] the sea was so choppy. We would have took a beating if we had gone full throttle." Ryan remembered it was "pretty rough" and they "caught some air" [the boat went into the air] on the way to the scene.

Most people involved in maritime search and rescue will admit that luck can play a large part in any rescue attempt.

D'Amelio and his crew arrived near the tip of the north jetty and came upon a "lull. It was breaking way outside, past [buoy] 7, so I could hug the jetty right in. . . . We cut right in [and] took fifteen- to eighteen-foot breaks. We had two guys [on the motor lifeboat] looking forward and two looking back for these people in the boat. Wham! The guy is right off our stern, about three hundred yards. Lucked out big time."

D'Amelio turned the 47-footer around and made an inbound run toward the 21-foot pleasure craft. "Squared up. Took four or five big breaks," he recalled. "I tried to back [the boat] in to get to them. It was taking way too long. There [were] four people hanging onto the hull of this boat. Getting pounded. So, we waited for those three or four breaks again [and] made another inbound run [and] got right up to them. Once we got to where they were, it was inside the jetty, so it was a little smaller. Second generation waves. We got up right alongside. As soon as we got alongside the helo came. They were on our port side, the boat is right in the middle of us. We got within ten feet."

The crew of the 47-foot motor lifeboat tried to coax the four people hanging onto the overturned boat to let go of it and swim over; if not, the lifesavers would throw them a line. Three of the four people in the water wore lifejackets; the owner of the boat did not. Perhaps not too surprisingly, all of the people in the water refused to let go of the overturned boat. Although the capsized boat was in a sheltered location, "they were still getting pounded."

Helicopter 6008 had arrived on scene with rescue swimmer Forslund on board. A "wall of water" knocked a survivor, who was not wearing a lifejacket, away from the hull of the overturned boat. Dennis DeWinter, the hoist operator, immediately began to lower Forslund into the water. The rescue swimmer did not leap into the water because the depth of the water was unknown and the because of the high surf conditions. Forslund swam to the survivor and then, using a cross chest carry, swam the man to the motor lifeboat.[17]

Petty Officer Slade recalled, "Chris was driving from the starboard seat. Normally he would have switched to the left seat, but he was talking on the radio and had so much going on, he stayed over there so he could talk to the helo." Slade remembered that "Petty Officer Ryan, myself, and Seaman [Owen] Corcran, just out of boot camp a week or two, [who] did not really know what was going on . . . [went down] into the recess. [Meanwhile,] Fireman Kibby stood on the port side . . . throwing the life ring."

Surfman D'Amelio later recalled that Fireman Kibby throwing the life ring "was relaying [information] to me on the starboard side. I could have jumped to the other side, but I would have had to unclip [my surf belt] and he would have had to unclip, and you never know what could happen. I could actually hear those guys down . . . [in the recess.] Your adrenalin is going and you're yelling loud. Normally, you can't hear from down there, but when your adrenaline is kicking, I could definitely hear them."

D'Amelio also explained that he did something "we do not train for: the [crew was] picking up the people, we were getting sluffing breaks. We were beam to and you could roll. . . . As soon as the wave was comin', and started sluffing a little bit, I'd actually pivot a little bit to port and get . . . knocked over a little bit." Surfman D'Amelio pointed out that instead of putting the bow into the breaking waves, known as "squaring up," as trained, the maneuver protected the crew from the breaks and helped them pick the people out of the water. "If I'd been squared, they'd have got hammered," he said. "When I got back, Mr. Burke said, 'I thought you were going to roll the boat.' If it had been a plunging break, I wouldn't have done that. If it's feathering a little bit, you can do that and stay out of trouble. It would push us over. I'd square back up. It'd push us over. I'd square back up."

As Surfman D'Amelio maneuvered the 47-footer, Slade said that Fireman Kibby would throw the life ring to the rescue swimmer, "pulling him over from the top" of the motor lifeboat. "Down in the recess, you knew a break was coming. You'd hear Kibby scream and then the sound of the engines as Chris pivoted the boat so the break would not hit us directly. He was protecting us with the bow of the boat."

Forslund swam back to the survivors. As he approached the second survivor, a huge wave broke over them and Forslund found himself driven beneath the sea. The sea tore his face mask "away from his face."[18] Forslund held tightly to the survivor and signaled for the motor lifeboat crew to throw a life ring.

The two remaining survivors shared one lifejacket. Forslund, with great effort, towed the two men toward the 47-foot motor lifeboat. Nearing the boat, the surf began pushing the three men too close to the pitching, rolling boat. Forslund managed to get the survivors away from the boat so they could be picked up.

Back on board the motor lifeboat, Surfman D'Amelio said that his crew "had the hardest job, picking up the [people in the water,] dealing with the lines, [and] the life rings. Physically, they had the toughest job."

"The first guy on board," recalled Slade, "was the smallest. By the time we got him, . . . he was limp, he was pretty much dead weight. We got him into the recess. Right when we got him into the recess, we got hit pretty good. [The breaker] filled the recess with water. [It] startled us a little bit. Ryan threw himself over the guy."

Ryan recalled it was "treacherous" in the recess. "Those waves were big and I had never been that close to the water and experienced taking breaks like that. Thank goodness for the surf-belts keeping you in the boat."

Slade explained, "It's hard [pulling] someone [from the water] when they're limp. It's such a small area in the recess. [You] have to unclip your belt and try to walk him up, [even] as you're dealing with the breaks. We got him onto the aft deck. He started foaming really bad, so Ryan stayed with him."

Ryan recalled, "I basically made sure the guy didn't fall off" the boat. "I took a pulse and didn't get anything. I took another and the guy moved. Then I tried again and could not get a pulse."

Surfman D'Amelio now had a difficult decision. The first person taken from the water needed medical attention. D'Amelio would have to exit the surf zone and move further out so the helicopter could lift him off the motor lifeboat. This meant he would have to leave the other three survivors in the water, getting beaten by the surf. In an understatement, D'Amelio said it "was a tough decision." D'Amelio took the only option available to him: he would retrieve the three in the water and then move out to have the helicopter take the first survivor off the motor lifeboat.

Slade recalled that "Corcran came back down to the recess deck with me and we got the other three guys. We had them lined up three in a row." The crew could not take the rescued men into the survivor's compartment, "as we couldn't break water tight integrity because of the breaks. We were pitching so badly that we did not want to send a crewman after the EMT kit, as that might have caused a crewman to become airborne." Slade remembered that everyone huddled "behind the towing bit. Ryan held the guy that was unconscious. Chris started to push out of the surf." Slade recalled that D'Amelio yelled back how was everyone? "I remember," said Slade, "Ryan yelling, 'What do I do?' He'd checked for a pulse and couldn't find [one.]"

As D'Amelio and his crew worked to get all the survivors on board, the motor lifeboat was "getting pushed into the jetty. We were probably fifty to seventy-five yards from the jetty, which really looks close when you're out there, especially when you've got breaking waves all around you." Even while battling the waves, maneuvering the 47-footer and monitoring what was taking place on the deck aft of him, D'Amelio talked with the rescue helicopter. "I talked to the helo saying we need to get this guy off. They're saying, yeah, you're right, but we can't do it in here. The plan was to go to the main channel, which was about one and one-half miles away. I decided to go straight west, go about a mile offshore where it [was] not breakin'. Get this guy off as fast as possible."

D'Amelio maneuvered the 47-footer the one and a half miles for the hoist. There was a eighteen-foot-long, rolling swell. "It was tough," he said. "You normally do helo ops when it's flat."

"Once we got out of the surf zone," Slade recalled, "we put the other three guys down below [in the survivor's compartment.] We also sent Corcran down there because he had never seen helo ops. There would be three guys on deck working and that's enough people. Corcran, God bless his heart, sat down there with a bucket, as some of the [survivors] were seasick. Corcran was not feeling very well himself, [but] he passed around the bucket, holding it for all these guys."

The helicopter lowered the rescue basket. "[We] put [the survivor] in the basket," recalled Slade. "It was tough to do, with none of us clipped in at that point. When the boat would go up, the basket would rise. We had to hold the basket to keep it from going off the stern. When the boat would drop, we had to wedge ourselves between the tow bit and push out so the basket would not fall on us. It felt like a long time on that deck, but it was probably only a few seconds." Surfman D'Amelio recalled that his crew "was dead tired, but it was the smoothest basket hoist I have ever done."

After the rescue helicopter flew the survivor to the north jetty, a waiting ambulance took him off to the hospital. Unfortunately, the man did not survive. The motor lifeboat brought the three other survivors to the station.

"From the time we left [the station] to the time we got back was about forty-five minutes," D'Amelio remembered. "We were in the surf about fifteen minutes, but it seemed much longer. It seemed about one to two hours." Much later, D'Amelio related the reason some boats end up in difficulties is that when the swells are running high, a boater can not see the buoys or the jetty. He pointed out that earlier on this same day, when he and his crew worked the case of the two men in Peacock Spit, as they exited the breaks, they saw a pleasure boat heading into the spit. The operator said, "Aren't we going to Ilwaco?" D'Amelio recalled that the U.S. Coast Guard crew told the operator to follow them. "There was a little kid on board. That's when you get a little mad and say, 'You've got to pay attention.'"

For their work on this rescue, Christopher D'Amelio received the Coast Guard Commendation Medal and a Gold Medal from the Association for Rescue at Sea. D'Amelio's boat crew received the Coast Guard Achievement Medal. Eric T. Forslund received the Coast Guard Meritorious Service Medal, with an operational device, and a Gold Medal from the Association for Rescue at Sea. This was the first time that the Association for Rescue at Sea had awarded their coveted Gold Medal to two people from different units for the same rescue. Dennis DeWinter received the Coast Guard Achievement Medal.[19]

WHALE STRIKE

Those who serve at U.S. Coast Guard stations can never tell what type of call they will receive. Not every case deals with a dramatic rescue in high seas, nor do all U.S. Coast Guard personnel receive medals for responding to distress calls. Take, for example, the events at Morro Bay, California, in 2002. At 6:30 P.M. on Sunday, 1 September, on another busy Labor Day holiday weekend, the communications watchstander at Station Morro Bay, California, received a Mayday call reporting a person in the water ten nautical miles south of Morro Bay. Six minutes later, the 47-foot motor lifeboat CG-47280 sped from the station's moorings, followed closely by the station's other motor lifeboat and a fast rigid hull boat.[20]

At the best of times, a person in the water can be difficult to locate. The weather made this case doubly difficult. Winds were light and seas at no more than one foot, but the visibility was twenty-five yards in dense fog.

Four minutes after the 47-footer departed, the watchstander received a cell telephone call from a "distraught" person on board the 22-foot white-and-blue pleasure craft *BBQ*. The person calling said the man in the water was from *BBQ*. While maneuvering through the thick fog, a whale had breached and rolled down the side of the craft, throwing Jerry Tibbs, the owner and operator of the boat, into the water without a lifejacket on. The three remaining passengers immediately began to throw lifejackets and anything that would float into the water. Tibbs "was conscious and appeared to have suffered no injuries when he hit the water," but he quickly disappeared from view in the fog. The passengers did not know how to obtain their position for rescuers. Like many passengers in pleasure craft, they were not paying attention to their location. They did remember, however, that Tibbs had said they were ten nautical miles out of Morro Bay. None of the passengers knew how to turn on or operate the GPS equipment on board the boat. Then the passengers made another chilling discovery: the whale had split the hull of *BBQ* and water was entering the 22-footer. Only one lifejacket remained on board.

Pleasure craft, harbor patrols, a California Highway Patrol helicopter, and U.S. Coast Guard small boats, helicopters, and a fixed-wing aircraft groped their way in the fog, attempting to locate *BBQ*. Despite the heavy fog, within forty-eight minutes after receiving the Mayday broadcast, CG-47231, with Boatswain's Mate 1st Class John Rose as coxswain, arrived at *BBQ*'s location. Chief Boatswain's Mate Michael Saindon, officer in charge of Station Morro Bay and on board the rigid hull boat, radioed that the boat had half-inch cracks on its starboard side; the transom was also damaged, though there was "not a lot of water in the boat" as the bilge pumps were keeping up with the water. One of the U.S. Coast Guard boats took *BBQ* in tow to Port San Luis Obispo. EMTs treated two of the passengers for mild hypothermia and then released the survivors, while the remaining passenger "suffered contusions on his head and had severe hypothermia" and was taken to a hospital for treatment. Back at Station Morro Bay, when Jerry Tibbs's wife, Patty, learned her husband was the person who "had fallen overboard, she collapsed and required medical attention." Chief Saindon and his crew began an immediate search for Tibbs. Thirty-eight minutes after starting the search, the crew found a sock, but nothing else.

The search for Tibbs continued throughout the night. At 12:50 P.M. on Monday, 2 September, the pleasure craft *Death Wish* located the body of Jerry Tibbs.

GOD WAS WITH US

The people who work in maritime search and rescue rarely have cases that are an uncomplicated "I'm in trouble, come and get me" coupled with an accurate position. It can be difficult sorting out conflicting information and coming up with a successful rescue. Sometimes the contradictory flow of data can lead to disastrous results. With training, and luck, this does not often happen. A rescue by the crew of the station at Erie, Pennsylvania, is a good example of success, despite a large flow of differing data from various sources.

Emil Michalaczik and James McCoure decided to go fishing on Monday night, 7 July 2003. They rented a 14-foot aluminum boat and headed out into Lake Erie. After a while, the "lake kicked up quite a bit," said Michalaczik. He started back to the boat rental dock. As their boat splashed through the choppy lake, McCoure moved to the side of the boat where Michalaczik sat, placing all the weight on one side of the small boat. At just this time, a wave struck and threw both men into the lake. Michalaczik later recalled that "the motor stayed running at full idle, doing circles and almost hitting us." Neither Michalaczik nor McCoure were wearing lifejackets.[21]

As fate would have it, two other men, Brian Emerick and Brad Watson, in a 12-foot boat, saw the capsized rental craft. They fired three flares and then went to help the two men struggling in the water. Instead, the boat carrying the would-be rescuers capsized and threw Emerick and Watson into the lake.[22]

A third party in another boat saw a capsized boat and a flare but did not go to the area. Instead, the person returned to harbor and called Station Erie on the radio, via channel 16, the international calling and distress frequency.[23]

Erie Station's SAR case folder records that at 8:40 P.M. they received a call of one "red flare straight off of Twelve Mile Creek, [and that the reporting source saw] the boat lite off flare." The caller said there were two people on board the boat firing the flares. The source said he could not help the people, "so he went back to boat launch and call[ed] Coast Guard."[24] Shortly after that, another citizen also notified the station of seeing a flare from the shore.

The U.S. Coast Guard receives many reports every year of flare sightings. Usually, they turn out to be false alarms, but the response to the calls is immediate. The station's communications watchstander briefed the station's OD (officer of the day) and the group. Five minutes after receiving the radio call, the watchstander issued an urgent marine broadcast that reported three red flares "in the vicinity of [Twelve] Mile Creek." The broadcast requested all vessels to keep a sharp watch, "assist if possible and report all sightings to the United States Coast Guard."

Ten minutes after receiving the call, Erie Station's 47-foot motor lifeboat, CG-47241, and a crew made up of Boatswain's Mate 3d Class Jeffery Jobczynski, the coxswain, Machinery Technician 2d Class Jonathan Moreno, the boat engineer, and crewmen Boatswain's Mate 3d Class Brandon McComas, Fireman Apprentice Shawn Vandenberg, and Seaman Apprentice Robert Paulino Jr. left the dock en route to the flare sighting area, eight nautical miles from the station.

The group duty officer of Group Buffalo, New York, could not at first contact the reporting source by telephone. In the meantime, the 47-footer arrived on scene. Once in the area, the crew of the 47-footer reported the weather as three-foot seas, winds from 350 degrees at ten knots. The lifesavers also reported finding no trace of any capsized boat. Coxswain Jobczynski started a shoreline search east to the New York state line, sixteen nautical miles to the east of the station. During the first leg of the search, "an unidentified woman reported earlier seeing a vessel fitting the description of the search" drifting a mile to the west of Freeport Beach, some four and a half nautical miles east of Twelve Mile Creek. The woman caller estimated the boat at least a mile offshore.

The group duty officer made many telephone calls trying to contact the person reporting the flares. Eventually, the duty officer located and quizzed the person about the flares and location of the sightings. One method used by the service to handle flare sightings is to question the reporting source on the angle of elevation of the flares. For inexperienced people on the water, and most people fall into this category, the U.S. Coast Guard has a form that helps in locating the position of the flares. Since most people on the water are inexperienced, the form instructs search personnel to ask the person reporting the sighting "to hold his/her arm at arm's length, make a fist, and place the bottom of the fist on the horizon. If the elevation of the flare is ABOVE the fist, the angle is greater than

8 degrees. Any elevation above 8 degrees can be approximated as the distance to the flare is within 1 NM [nautical mile]. If the elevation is BELOW the top of the fist, ascertain how high up the fist, i.e., 1/4, 1/2, 3/4 or number of fingers. The distance to the source of the flare is much greater for any angle below 8 degrees." Conversion tables on the back of the form help in converting this to distance. In this case, the person reporting the flare estimated an angle of elevation of no less than ten degrees or more than twenty degrees, with an estimated sixteen degrees. Using the information from the form, searchers determined the distance to the flares from the reporting source was one-quarter nautical miles. In addition, once contacted, the reporting source said the flares bore 340 degrees from his location on the shore. The official report on the rescue stated that over the next thirty minutes "of very confusing information gathering, the reporting source was unable to confirm the location or status of the vessel."

At 9:45 P.M., Station Erie received a telephone report of a 14-foot boat, with two people on board, which set out to look for the first boat and never returned. The communications watchstander notified the 47-foot crew that they were now searching for two missing boats and, possibly, four people in the water. A friend of one of the missing men called the U.S. Coast Guard. She said that the people in both boats knew one another and they normally fished near Sand Cliffs, "which is geographically between [Twelve] Mile Creek and Freeport Beach." The group duty officer and Rescue Coordination Center of the Ninth District, in Cleveland, Ohio, decided to place their search efforts in this area. Both had agreed that the newly reported overdue boat was either the actual boat the 47-footer was searching for or it "was attempting to assist their friends." The group duty officer drafted search plans for aircraft and the 47-footer in the area.

At 10:50 P.M., Coxswain Jobczynski, near Sand Cliffs, requested permission to fire a MK-127 illumination flare. The parachute flare puts out 125,000 candlepower of illumination. Jobczynski's crew continued to light off flares. At 11:51, the fourth flare sent down its cold, white light. Two minutes later, the communications watchstander received a radio call from the 47-footer that they had a visual sighting of two people in the water. One minute after this radio message, the watchstander received the radio report from the motor lifeboat crew that they had a total of four people in the water holding onto an overturned boat. Two of the four people were in lifejackets and two were not wearing flotation devices. At 11:59, the watchstander logged that all four people in the water were on board the motor lifeboat, suffering from mild hypothermia. The 47-footer shaped a course for Erie, while requesting medical personnel meet them at the docks. Forty-four minutes later, at 12:43 A.M., after dropping off the four survivors, the motor lifeboat moored at Station Erie. The official chronological log of the incident records that the total time the crew of CG-47241 took to save four lives was three hours and forty-three minutes.[25]

Later, Michalaczik told reporter Tim Hahn of the *Erie Times-News* that the experience "was very scary, but God was with us. . . . He was."[26]

14 | Helicopters versus Gales

The aviation branch of the U.S. Coast Guard entered the twenty-first century employing two main helicopters in search and rescue: the HH-60A Jayhawk and the HH-65A Dolphin. The rescues in this chapter illustrate the use of these helicopters and prove once again that aviation crews show the same dedication and valor as their predecessors in the service.

LORD, YOU GOTTA MAKE THIS HAPPEN

Cdr. Paul A. Langlois woke to the ringing of the telephone in the senior duty officer's quarters of the U.S. Coast Guard Air Station Port Angeles, Washington, shortly before 1:00 A.M. on 12 February 1997. A Mayday radio call had been received from the sailboat *Gale Runner.* Langlois told the duty officer to hit the SAR alarm and provide the ready helicopter with the rescue swimmer and night vision goggles. Then Langlois climbed into his survival suit and made his way to the station's operations center. *Gale Runner* had first given its position as crossing the dangerous bar on the Quillayute River at LaPush, Washington. Then came a message that the boat was taking on water. Langlois hurried to the helicopter.[1]

239

Aviation Survivalman 1st Class Charles "Chuck" Carter, the rescue swimmer, still fighting off sleep, arrived at helicopter 6589 and joined copilot Cdr. Raymond J. Miller and Aviation Structural Mechanic 3d Class Neal Amos, the flight mechanic and rescue winch operator. Sailboats on the Northwest Coast in February are rare, and the weather was so foul there was discussion as to whether this might be a hoax. (The U.S. Coast Guard received 729 hoaxes from 1994 to 1996.) As the helicopter started, and before Langlois arrived, over the radio came the information that two 44-foot motor lifeboats from the U.S. Coast Guard Quillayute River Station had responded, but the station had lost communications with both boats. Carter later recalled, "I was instantly awake. I went from thinking this is a hoax to thinking I had *ten* people in the water. Commander Miller over the radio was going: 'Call the commanding officer.' He made a bunch of other commands, and then he said, 'Gentlemen, this is the real thing!'"

Commander Langlois arrived and gave his crew a briefing. Helicopter 6589 departed Port Angeles at 1:18 A.M. The helicopter began to run into low clouds and moderate rain with strong southwest winds. "Flying direct to the scene," recalled Langlois, "over the [Olympic] mountains would have been a shorter distance, but was too dangerous due to potential icing conditions, probable turbulence, and high terrain in instrument conditions." Instead, the pilots elected to fly along the Strait of Juan de Fuca to Tatoosh Island and then turn south along the coast to the Quillayute River area staying over water.

Langlois flew the helicopter between five hundred and eight hundred feet off the water. Cockpit instruments registered a temperature of thirty-four degrees Fahrenheit and winds from the southwest at forty knots during the leg from Port Angeles to Tatoosh Island. "We were picking up a little ice on the helicopter and gusts were up to 60 knots," recalled Langlois. "We took quite a beating over the strait. The winds were from the southwest and they tend to spin off the mountains to cause turbulence and that causes a rough ride, which causes the pucker factor to go up." The weather caused an instrument flight all the way to the Quillayute

River area. "We flew at maximum performance," said Langlois, "which gave us about 140 knots indicated airspeed." Langlois flew the helicopter while Commander Miller quickly became comfortable with the night vision goggles, handled the communications and backed up the pilot in command with navigation.

"Our attention and focus had shifted from the sailboat to the grim reality that our own motor lifeboat might be in distress," said Langlois. "We all privately hoped the motor lifeboat had just lost their comms, and were otherwise all right."

Turning onto the southbound leg at Tatoosh Island, the winds were forty knots, with some gusts to fifty-three knots. The pilots heard a "very scared" female voice on the radio give a precise latitude and longitude of *Gale Runner*'s position. "I suspected she had GPS [global positioning system]," said Langlois. "I envisioned that we would be able to easily locate the sailboat and not have to search after we first located the motor lifeboat with the lost comms."

"We knew one of the 44s was in the water and so when we got on scene we had a question," said Carter. "Do we look for the Coast Guard people in the water, or do we go to the people on the boat? I heard Commander Miller discussing this decision. You think, 'Wow, this is a really tough decision.' You got Coast Guard people who might be dying and you got civilian people who might be dying."

Approximately thirty-nine minutes after liftoff from Port Angeles, the rescue helicopter arrived near James Island, just off LaPush. Langlois shifted his view from the instruments to the outside and quickly viewed the lights of LaPush. He spotted the second motor lifeboat, the CG-44393, driven by Boatswain's Mate 1st Class Jonathan Placido, near the Quillayute River sea buoy. Langlois later recalled the spotlight of the motor lifeboat, which normally would be tracking at the horizon, "was going in oscillations of almost straight down to vertical. I could tell from Placido's voice [on the radio] that he was not enjoying the situation he was in. I then realized how high the seas must have been."

Langlois descended to approximately 300 feet and slowed to 70 knots. He discussed with Miller about staying on the night vision goggles. Langlois knew the rugged coastline. The wind direction would push the helicopter toward the east and into the offshore rocky spires and cliffs. Miller agreed to keep on the night-vision goggles.

Langlois, as the pilot in command, briefed his crew that they were searching for Quillayute River's ready lifeboat, the CG-44363, before going to the assistance of the sailboat. He would fly the aircraft on instruments, while Miller would control the heading with the heading knob located on the instrument panel near his right leg. Most important, with the night vision goggles, Miller would be able to better see the towering rock spires, known as the "Needles."

After several minutes of searching for the motor lifeboat, the pilots heard Master Chief Boatswain's Mate George A. LaForge, the officer in charge of the Quillayute River Station, on the radio. The master chief made a difficult decision: he recommended Langlois break off the search for the missing CG-44363, as his navigation plot indicated the sailboat was drifting rapidly toward the Needles. Later, Miller said, "Our entire crew found it very difficult to interrupt our search for the 44363."

Langlois turned the helicopter toward the last reported position of *Gale Runner*. A few minutes later, the helicopter crew spotted a dim light ahead. Miller informed Langlois that he saw rock formations through the night vision goggles near the sailboat. The steep, towering rocks would interfere with their descent to a hover over the dismasted and out-of-control sailboat.

Langlois informed his crew they would do a basket recovery of the people aboard *Gale Runner*. The use of the rescue swimmer was too dangerous among the rocks. Langlois informed the other three crewmembers he would use instruments to make a letdown to a hover. Miller would stay on the night vision goggles continuously and give him any steering commands around the rocks, towering to 190 feet into the air, while he attempted to keep the helicopter pointed into the wind. Besides the wind and darkness, the helicopter flew through lashing horizontal rain.

Miller later recalled, "I could discern the rock formations of The Needles. I told Commander Langlois that we would have to work our way over and around some high rocks to get down where we needed to be to conduct a hoist." Miller continued on the night-vision goggles and controlling the heading, while advising Langlois of the descent rate. Through the night vision goggles, Miller could see *Gale Runner* to the west of the rocks and about three hundred yards away from them. Miller knew the helicopter would have to make a steep approach into the wind to clear the rocks safely and arrive at an altitude to hover near the sailboat. "I was comfortable on the night vision goggles. I'm not too sure how comfortable the crew was after I described the rocks.

"I could see the rocks very well," said Miller. The helicopter flew over and *between* the rocks, ending at 150 feet above *Gale Runner* and at sixty-five knots indicated airspeed. Too high and fast. Both pilots called for a "go around." The helicopter turned right and departed toward LaPush. The four U.S. Coast Guardsmen over the terror-filled minutes ahead would be dodging between rocks that rose to at least the height of a nineteen-story building.

Miller fine-tuned the approach and told Langlois when they had cleared the rocks. Langlois then descended very steeply and arrived at a seventy-five-foot altitude, with *Gale Runner* at their one-thirty position. The radar altimeter, which indicates altitude from the surface, so critical to the crew's safety, surged between seventy-five and thirty-five feet, a good indication of the height of the seas. Miller continued to scan the horizon with the night-vision goggles. *Gale Runner* moved wildly in the towering seas, almost broaching. Langlois briefed his crew on a trail line delivery.

Miller called the sailboat. "I instructed them to clear any downed rigging from the cockpit as best they could. I explained the trail line delivery of the rescue basket." Langlois also "instructed Petty Officer Carter to keep an active scan out his window to the back, and advise us when he saw the rocks." Langlois told Miller not to let him get below twenty-five feet over the wave tops. Flight mechanic Amos, talking through the helicopter's intercom system, gave Langlois instructions to guide him over *Gale Runner*. The wild movement of the sailboat and the battering wind prevented the helicopter from hovering over the wildly pitching and wallowing craft. "Neal certainly was doing his best at giving me conning commands," said Langlois. "We were both very frustrated. We couldn't maintain our position in relation to the boat."

Carter recalled, "We're trying to do the basket hoist and it's just not working. Neal said to Commander Langlois, 'You've gotta hold it steady.'

"Commander Langlois said, 'I am.'

"*'You're not doing it, sir!'*

"It was just frustration. Everybody was frustrated."

Trying to make the hoist work, Langlois *backed* the helicopter through the gale-swept night. The aircraft moved closer and closer to the rock pinnacles. "None of us were absolutely sure what obstructions were directly behind us," said Langlois. "My focus continued with trying to get the people off the boat before they hit the rocks."

Carter said, "In the light from the helicopter's search light I can remember the boat coming up and dropping down the backside of a wave. It looked like they fell off the face of the earth. You could see them. Then they were gone."

Langlois recalled that Amos said the trail line was streaming straight back in the wind, despite the weight bags. "I told him to get rid of the trail line. Let's see if we could just put the basket on deck directly." Langlois said that "throughout the whole hovering sequence, Ray was giving me incredibly precise advisories on power, altitude, and whatever he could see through his night vision goggles." Then Langlois suffered from vertigo. Miller helped keep the helicopter steady. At one point, Langlois shifted his scan to the limited view to the rear of the helicopter. "I saw a large rock pinnacle right behind our aircraft at the five o'clock position. . . . Carter thankfully alerted me to the rock." The rock was higher than the altitude of the helicopter. "I have to admit I got pretty scared at that point," Langlois said, "and now fully realized the danger in which I had placed the whole aircrew." Then

Langlois related something most people in maritime search and rescue eventually say: "I'm sure I became reliant on adrenalin and instinct to continue the effort." He continued to try to get the basket onto *Gale Runner,* but to no avail.

Carter said, "We've gotta do something different. They said, 'What?' I said, 'Put me down.' [They said,] 'We can't do that. It'll kill you.' I really didn't want to go down, but we were at the point of what else are we goin' to do? I said, 'We've gotta do something.' At that point, we had the basket inside and Commander Langlois said, 'There's nothing we can do.' And I thought, *We're the United States Coast Guard!* If there's nothing we could do, then who could do anything? I remembered I just started praying, 'Lord, if you're out there, you gotta make this happen.'

"I thought for sure they were going to die. We were going to sit there and watch those people die. The concept that we couldn't help someone never entered my mind. I mean, we can't do anything is not the right answer.

"There was this huge rock. The sailboat was coming at this huge rock. I expected them to hit the rock and they would explode. I thought this boat was just going to be gone."

Recalled Langlois, "I remember this was the most challenging, stressful, frustrating time I've ever had flying—ever! I have always been able to make a rescue, this time I could not do it. As each minute went by, *Gale Runner* was getting closer and closer to the rocks. Rocks were behind us and higher than the helicopter. I told Ray I could not do this.

"Ray could see that the boat was now approaching some rocks immediately north of The Needles. The surf was getting even bigger, with waves starting to break, completely engulfing the boat. Ray called on the radio and told them they only had a few seconds to get in the cabin and brace for impact with the rocks. Over the next minute, the sailboat was repeatedly swamped in tremendous curling waves, which made the boat disappear from sight for periods of three to five seconds at a time. Judging from the size of the 31-foot sailboat, I would estimate the breaking waves must have easily been thirty feet. We all privately knew that the people could surely not survive that thrashing. Finally, the boat ended up being tossed on a rock shelf above the surface, laying on its side. By now, I had the Needles directly in front of me, as we had maneuvered clear around it. I remained very concerned that there may be other obstructions right behind us, but not in sight."

Miller recalls "telling the people on the boat they had sixty seconds before you crash on the rocks. Go below and prepare yourself." Ken Schlag and Maria Infante, the two people on *Gale Runner,* went below. "I looked through the goggles and could see a narrow gap between the one large spire and the smaller shelf the boat was lying on. As each wave was coming against the windward shore, there was this like flushing funnel of water that would go through this narrow gap. Sure enough, their boat was being sucked toward it. As I sat there, I thought to myself, 'Nature has a chance of pulling them through there.'

"Sure enough! The sailboat went right through there. It pitch-poled. It went over and it went under and completely out of sight like a submarine for a short while, for a matter of seconds. It seemed a lot longer to us. Then up it came. After it washed through, breakers were coming through the shelf and the boat got pushed upon another shelf behind the outer rocks and landed on its side. So there it sat, high and dry. A few waves came over it, but not enough to push it over. So we thought. There was a lull between the series. Through the goggles I could see the boat on its side, the cabin lights were still on and I could see people moving in there. I thought, 'They made it through this. They might just be able to climb right out of the cabin. There they are on the shelf and all of a sudden there was this chance for us to scoot over there and pick them up off this rock.'

"No sooner had I thought that and uttered it to the crew, than the next series came through. The boat was on its side with the keel facing toward the sea. The next series came through and got underneath that keel and lifted the whole boat over into deep water on the shore side of the rock and under it went again. It popped right back up. This time it popped up right side up, stern to the waves. It was past three pretty good sized rocks that were moderating the action of the waves, so the boat was still moving around, but it wasn't impossible like it was on the seaward side."

By this time, Langlois had been flying the helicopter in horrible weather for over an hour, including the time to reach the Needles. "As worn out as I was at this point," Langlois recalled, "I said to Ray and the flight mechanic, 'I think we might be able to continue to try to do this. Let's keep trying.'"

Miller related, "So very carefully, and here again is where the night vision goggles paid off, rather than take off in forward flight with the basket hanging out, which you really can not do, we kind of picked our way, back and around and got into position right next to the boat. From there on out, it was a matter of only five minutes until we had both people in the helicopter. Paul Langlois did an amazing job after being so drained from all the effort offshore.

"We turned sideways so I could see. I said, 'Come left 50 feet. You're clear of the rocks. Watch out you don't get behind the rocks.' With the wind blowing at 40 knots, rocks create a lot of turbulence. You want to stay clear of those zones because that can put you in the water before you can blink.

"We were about 150–200 feet from the rocks. It always looks closer when you are in a situation like that." Miller would later remember that throughout the long fight, "I was constantly reminding myself that this is for real. We can do this. It was like there was a self-generated pep rally going on in my head, or a checklist.

"Are we at the outer limits? No. Check!

"Can we do this? Yes. Check!

"Okay, we're still okay.

"I'm still alive. Check!

"They're still alive. Check!

"Every minute or two, this test. We actually yanked them off the sailboat. We stressed the hoist so much the mounting brackets had to be replaced."

"Neal did an incredible job of commanding me," recalled Langlois. "Neal said the lady is getting into the basket. We dragged the basket down one side of the boat and it snagged. I remember a pretty good tension on the hoist. The basket broke free and came up almost like a pendulum, almost high enough to strike the rotor. I've never seen a basket swing like that before.

Carter remembered looking down at *Gale Runner* as it shot through the gap in the Needles. "They were completely gone. It was, like, they're gone! They're back! There they are!

"We backed all the way around those needles and I can't really see anything out there. We did the two hoists lickety-split. First she came up and then him. I was so amazed they didn't both come up at the same time. After all we'd been through, I know I wouldn't have waited for another hoist. Come to find out, they were both pretty small people. Weight wise we could have picked them both up.

"They're in the plane and I'm, like, 'How're you doing?'

"'We're fine.'

"They both looked fine, they weren't bleeding and nothing was broken. I didn't even have time to give them a blanket."

"We all took a big breath," recalled Langlois. "I said, 'Ray, let's get out of here.' I was completely drained, both mentally and physically. It was the hardest thing I ever did in a helicopter."

Much later, Commander Langlois recalled, "We all believed something miraculous helped us. Somebody above was watching over us. There must have been enough pain in losing our own crew that somehow it was right to help those two people." (Three U.S. Coast Guardsmen were lost in the first motor lifeboat.)

Cdr. Raymond J. Miller said the battle to save the two people from *Gale Runner* gave "an heightened sense of being connected to the process. In a way it comes from fear and fueled by adrenalin. It is a very invigorating experience, too. Not that you would ever want to buy a ticket and do it again, not on purpose anyway. There is that sense at the end of it of gratification, not pride, but, my goodness! look at what people and machines can do when they really have to."

For their work, Paul A. Langlois, Raymond J. Miller, and Neal Amos received the Distinguished Flying Cross. This was the second Distinguished Flying Cross awarded to Miller. Charles

Carter received the U.S. Coast Guard Commendation Medal with operational device. Carter later said that he felt he received the medal for sitting in the aircraft and "praying a lot."

DO I REALLY HAVE TO DIE COLD AND WET?

The fishing vessel *La Conte* battled towering seas 65 nautical miles offshore in the Gulf of Alaska, 120 miles northwest of Sitka. On board the vessel was Mark Morley, the captain, and his crew of Robert Doyle, Gig Mork, Michael DeCapua, and David Hanlon. The wooden fishing vessel measured seventy-seven feet and was nearly eighty years old. Seas of at least fifty feet slammed into it, and winds gusted between fifty and seventy knots. Visibility was fifty feet, and the wind chill was minus eighteen degrees Fahrenheit. Sea temperature measured a mere thirty-nine degrees. As *La Conte*'s bow shuddered slowly upward from yet another blow, a crewman yelled to Mark Morley, "Skipper. We got jeopardy!"[2]

Water rose in the engine room. The pumps failed. Morely ordered his crew into their survival suits, then they went into the engine room and bailed. Water rose to their necks. Morley looked down into the engine space and ordered the men to prepare to abandon *La Conte*. He went to the cabin to sent out a Mayday broadcast. Only static came back. Morley grabbed an electronic position indicating radio beacon (EPIRB). The device, about the size of a bowling pin, is activated by water if a vessel goes down. Morley tied his crew of five together with a three-quarter-inch line and at the end of the line attached two buoy floats and the EPIRB. There was no life raft. The men entered the furious sea.

At 7:02 P.M. on 30 January 1998, the U.S. Coast Guard's North Pacific Search and Rescue Coordination Center in Juneau, Alaska, received a message from the U.S. Mission Control Center, Suitland, Maryland, which relays EPIRB signals. The rescue center relayed the position of the EPIRB signal to Air Station Sitka, the unit closest to the signal.[3]

Lt. William Adickes, of U.S. Coast Guard Air Station Sitka, took off into the stormy night. As Adickes and his crew of Jayhawk

6018 moved out onto his flight path, they encountered buffeting seventy-knot winds. Adickes wondered, "How bad is this going to get?"[4] Lieutenant Adickes and his crew of 6018 flew in the U.S. Coast Guard's most powerful helicopter. The 21,246-pound machine pitched up and down at least one hundred feet, while flying at an altitude of three hundred feet. Fifty minutes after takeoff, Adickes's direction finder received a weak signal from the EPIRB. The directional finder showed the signal came from below them. The wind pushed the pitching and yawing aircraft past the position. With engines at full throttle, and "intense concentration and focus" by the two pilots, 6018 came to a one-hundred-foot hover near the people in the water.[5]

For the next hour, battling against winds that reached gusts of 120 knots, Adickes and his crew tried to pull *La Conte*'s crew from the sea. At one time the winds blew the helicopter backward half a mile. The rescue basket was continually blown away from the men in the water, and due to the constant hoisting attempts, the cable began to fray from rubbing against the aircraft. Squatting in the doorway in the back of the aircraft, rescue swimmer Richard Sansone and flight mechanic Sean Witherspoon looked up. There was the mind-numbing vision of a wave of at least one hundred feet in height. The white crest of the hissing wave was higher than the aircraft.[6]

In the water, the fishermen could scarcely believe their eyes. The helicopter was at least "thirty feet below them." They found themselves staring *down* at the Jayhawk's whirling blades.[7]

"Up! Up! Up! *Emergency Up!*" yelled Sansone over the intercom. "Altitude! Up! Up! Up! Take her up! *Now!*"[8]

The two pilots watched as the huge wave approached them. Both pilots grabbed their collective sticks alongside their seats and yanked up on them.

A downdraft prevented the Jayhawk from climbing. Four-thousand shaft horsepower screamed to make the helicopter climb. Slowly, slowly the Jayhawk moved upward. The wave washed five feet beneath the struggling helicopter. Writer Spike

Walker believes an Alaskan williwaw, a sudden fierce narrow blast of wind, struck the aircraft.[9]

No sooner had the Jayhawk cleared the wave than another fierce blast struck it. Unbelievably, the helicopter "rocketed backward."[10] Lieutenant Adickes feared the tail rotor would slam into a wave, spelling the deaths of the crew. He regained control of the helicopter and said over the intercom, "Okay, we need to regroup here. We need to retreat for a few minutes and get everybody calmed down."[11]

The helicopter crew continued their attempt. They expended their water-activated flares. The pilots heard over the intercom that Witherspoon was hypothermic.

Since arrival on scene, Adickes had had no communication. Then he gained radio contact with an Alaska Airlines commercial jet and passed on the situation to both Juneau and the second helicopter en route from Sitka to the scene.

Witherspoon began shaking and throwing up. After eighty minutes of attempted rescue, with their fuel dangerously low, a crewman in need of medical attention, and poor communications, Adickes finally said over the intercom system, "It's time to go."[12]

Following normal operating procedures, a backup helicopter, the 6029 from Sitka, started toward the scene at 9:35 P.M. Lt. Cdr. David Durham's only communications with the first helicopter was from the Alaskan Airlines commercial jet.[13]

Ten minutes after Adickes departed, the second helicopter arrived on scene. Durham saw survivors and the strobe light of the EPIRB. Flight mechanic Chris Windnagle put out three flares. He then attempted to lower the rescue basket. It blew back to near the tail of the helicopter. Windnagle could get the basket into the water close to the survivors, the closest he could set the basket was twenty feet from the weakening fishermen.[14] The inconsistency of the wave pattern worked against Windnagle. High, confused seas came from all directions. Durham tried to hold a hundred-foot hover. He had to continually gain altitude to let wave crests pass beneath them.

Meanwhile, in the water, *La Conte*'s crew now numbered four: David Hanlon had slipped from the line keeping the fishermen together and was lost. Morley was weakening. Numbing sea water entered through a rip in his survival suit. The survivors had now spent six hours fighting for their lives.[15]

Above the raging sea, the helicopter searched for the survivors. Once the pilots spotted the EPIRB light, they maneuvered the helicopter toward the location. Windnagle's voice came over the pilot's headset: "I've got four survivors in the water. I see four."[16]

Windnagle started lowering the rescue basket. It blew under the tail portion of the aircraft. Over the next hour and a half, and dozens of approaches, Windnagle continued to try to reach the survivors. At one time, the aircraft flew backward, tail down, close to eighty miles per hour.[17] Durham watched the last of the aircraft's flares sputter out. As the flares died out, Durham knew his fuel was critical; he had to break off the rescue attempt.

Back at Sitka, the air station's last Jayhawk, number 6011, was prepared for flight. Even though communications were bad, pilot Lt. Stephen Torpey realized he would need extra flares; he had his crew cram in thirty instead of the normal four. The crew also tied chemical lights to the rescue basket so the survivors could better see the basket. Also loaded were extra weight bags for the basket. Torpey elected to take an extra flight mechanic to help with the hoisting. He lifted off at 12:15 A.M., with a crew of Cdr. Ted Le Feuvre, copilot; Avionics Technician 1st Class Fred Kalt; Aviation Machinist Mate Lee Honnold; and Aviation Survivalman 2d Class Mike Fish.[18]

Torpey later recalled that "what helped me was being the third aircraft, and understanding a little better what I was up against."[19] Once on scene and able to see the seas they would face, Torpey and Le Feuvre felt the waves were the worse they had seen in thirty-two years of combined U.S. Coast Guard experience.[20]

The crew in the back of the aircraft found themselves thrown about in the darkened interior of the helicopter. "I experienced intense vertigo, like being spun around and around in a circle and then abruptly stopped," said rescue swimmer Mike Fish.[21] The pilots tried to maintain a hundred-foot hover. They fought an aircraft being flung sideways and up and down. Conditions made it virtually impossible to see the water. When they did see it, the helicopter was frighteningly close to the water. At times the 6011 was only thirty feet from the mountainous seas. When Le Feuvre came close to the breaking waves, he thought, "OK Lord, here I come. I'm gonna die. But do I really have to die cold and wet?"[22]

Later, Torpey admitted everyone's fright. He felt he had an advantage, however: "I had the stick in my hand, so I felt more control. But for the guys in the back, it was like being in a two-hour car crash. I felt badly for them. For me, I had a constant knot in the pit of my stomach. My concentration was very, very intense. I knew that any unexpected variable, however slight, could put the aircraft into a bad situation."[23]

The crew of 6011 had another advantage over the first two helicopters. A U.S. Coast Guard four engine, fixed wing C-130 aircraft from Kodiak arrived overhead to act as their communications link.[24]

In the midst of terrible conditions, Le Feuvre, to help take the entire burden of flying the aircraft off Torpey, suggested dividing the controls. He would work the collective, which would keep them at a safe altitude. Torpey would handle the stick and main controls and actually fly the helicopter.[25]

In the back of the Jayhawk, Kalt and Honnold battled unsuccessfully for an hour trying to lower the rescue basket close to the weakening survivors. It took the combined efforts of both men to keep the cable from shearing. Fish volunteered to go into the sea, but Torpey deemed it too risky. Two hours of battling finally brought the basket within a few feet of the survivors.

Torpey gained more and more confidence. At last came a chance. Kalt conned Torpey over the men. "Back and left fifty," came Kalt's voice in Torpey's headset. Between each command a pause, then, "Forward and right twenty. . . . Forward and right ten. . . . Now over top. Hold position. Preparing to take the load.

Taking the load. Basket is clear of the waves. Clear to move back and left thirty, sir."[26]

Up the basket came. Kalt could not see what was in it, as an auxiliary fuel tank and poor visibility blocked the view. Then Kalt saw one man in the basket. Both Kalt and Honnold struggled to get the basket in the door. The basket seemed heavier than normal. Then Fish yelled, "Fred! Someone's hanging on the basket."

Kalt yelled, "I can't see him."[27]

The person clinging to the basket could not hold on; he fell through the darkness into the sea. Rescuers pulled fisherman Robert Doyle into the helicopter. Doyle had entered the rescue basket, but the skipper of *La Conte,* Mark Morley, could not make it and had grabbed onto the basket.[28]

When the helicopter crew visually located Morely, he was floating face down. Torpey said, "We didn't give up on him, but I knew he couldn't have survived that fall."[29] Torpey concentrated his efforts on bringing the other two survivors aboard.

Fisherman Mike DeCapua and Gig Mork entered the basket. Just as the basket broke free of the sea, another wave hit them, throwing DeCapua back into the sea.[30] "Somebody else fell," said Honnald over the intercom. "A wave hit him."[31]

With two survivors aboard and two left in the water, another critical decision entered the mix. Facing strong headwinds on their return, the helicopter had to depart immediately from the scene if they were to make it back safely to Sitka. To gain additional time on scene, Torpey decided to land at Yakutat, about seventy miles closer to Sitka. This gave the rescue crew an extra hour. Kalt and Honnold lowered the basket and managed to bring up Mike DeCapua and Mork.[32]

Kalt recalled, "We tried to get Morley until fuel became a factor. We all knew he was gone." Honnold remarked, "We put the basket next to him and gave him every opportunity to get into it." Torpey, knowing the condition of the hoist cable, decided against putting Fish into the water.[33]

The first Jayhawk that had returned to Sitka had refueled and started toward the scene. When they realized there were no survivors, they turned for Sitka. Searchers in another Jayhawk recovered Morley's body the next day after the storm abated. David Hanlon's body remained missing until August 1998, seven months after the sinking of *La Conte*. Currents in the Gulf of Alaska carried Hanlon's body 650 miles to a remote location on Shuyak Island. Those on scene found most of Hanlon's body had been devoured by a bear. The three survivors recovered completely.[34]

For their amazing work in rescuing three of the five crewmen aboard *La Conte,* the entire crew of Jayhawk 6011, Stephen Torpey, Ted Le Feuvre, Fred Kalt, Lee Honnold, and Michael Fish, received the Distinguished Flying Cross and other honors. The other crews received commendation medals.[35] Although Lt. Stephen Torpey's crew received the highest aviation award for bravery in peacetime, Torpey summed up what everyone involved in the rescue felt: "I never want to go through something like that again."[36]

Epilogue

For more than 125 years, crews of the U.S. Coast Guard and one of its predecessors, the U.S. Life-Saving Service, have rammed small boats into large seas to help those in distress. The basic rescue mission has changed very little since 1878. Simply put, crews in small boats push out to help those in danger of losing their lives at sea. True, the equipment has changed and lifesavers from the early U.S. Life-Saving Service could hardly foresee a time when crews in aircraft could pluck people from the sea, yet the man-against-the-sea nature of shore-based maritime rescue has not changed. At times, the crews were successful, and at other times, the sea took lives. Crews won enough times so that most Americans look upon the U.S. Coast Guard as the premier maritime rescue organization of the United States. The rescue stories in this book show why this perception is true.

The lifesavers have managed to win the title of "experts" despite overwhelming odds against them—odds not only from the sea but also from their own service. One of the largest obstacles concerns a little-known fact of the U.S. Coast Guard. Very few people in the service carry the burden of search and rescue. While many officers and enlisted people say they are lifesavers, service statistics show it is the small boat rescue stations that largely undertake the business of maritime rescue. From 1986 to 2003, of the 84,019 lives saved by all units within the U.S. Coast Guard, 38,057 people owe their lives to those who serve at the stations. To put this in perspective, as of July 2003, there were 39,000 people on active duty in the service, but only 5,964 served at 188 small boat stations.[1] To paraphrase Winston S. Churchill, never have so many who venture out upon the waters owed so much to so few.

Those who carry the SAR load, the station crews, consist largely of the service's enlisted force, some chief warrant officers, and a smattering of commissioned officers.[2] This has traditionally put the stations near the bottom of the organization's hierarchy for budget, equipment, and sufficient personnel to run the stations. The U.S. Coast Guard's fiscal year 2002 budget request shows that search and rescue ranks fourth in priorities, with law enforcement, aids to navigation, and marine safety scheduled to receive more funding.[3] Crews often operate without state-of-the-art equipment and survival gear due to a lack of money.[4] In 1996, for example, a historian was given a ride in one of the then-new 47-foot motor lifeboats, and when he asked if it was difficult for the coxswain to hear people working lines at the towing bit, a coxswain and his training officer replied that it was, but the service was working on a method to improve communications between the two areas. As of July 2003, seven years later, there is still no improvement in communications between the two important areas.[5] Stations traditionally carried out their mission with very few people, which meant long hours of duty. Today, stations now have other missions along with SAR and are subject to frequent transfers of people, and, as always, crews struggle with long duty days. Additional missions and frequent transfers often leave units short of experienced people. After the *Mermaid* case, for example, newspapers revealed how the experience level of the crews on the Columbia River had dropped because of transfers. Yet thirty-six years later, the head of Boat Forces in Headquarters, the office responsible for stations, wrote in the United States Naval Institute *Proceedings* of the loss of experience level at the stations. While Washington, D.C., has a reputation for slowness, this borders on glacier-like movement.[6]

If the above were not enough, then the leadership's apparently strong desire to make the men and women who serve in the ranks anonymous can be discouraging. Very few people enjoy doing a good job without recognition for their contributions.

Finally, the current belief, especially in the media, is that if someone dies during a rescue attempt, the service, because it is the "expert," must have done something wrong. This leads to a feeling of discouragement among crews. The belief is not entirely the fault of the media, however. At the first word of deaths in any rescue attempt, members of the service are very quick to start pointing fingers. Mutterings abound that "it would not have happened if I had been in charge." Those who shove off into heavy weather to rescue someone must prepare themselves for the chance of censure, either rightly or wrongly, from their shipmates and the media. Further, there is anecdotal evidence to show that the people who do the most work in SAR, those at the stations, have a feeling that the leadership of the service cares little for what they accomplish. In other words, there is a disconnect between those who form policy and those who actually push out into an unforgiving environment to help others.[7]

People who perform the U.S. Coast Guard's search and rescue operations confront low funding, inferior equipment, a shortage of personnel, very little credit for what they accomplish, a feeling of being forgotten, sometimes harsh and unjust censure, and the chance of losing their lives in a rescue attempt. Given all this, why would anyone want to work in search and rescue?

Many in the service do not want to work in the field. Some transfer to the stations and quickly rotate out, swearing that if they have anything to say about it, they will never serve at another small boat station. Others do their allotted time at a unit and, though they do not hate their assignment, have no desire to ever return. There are others who think that duty at the stations is what separates the U.S. Coast Guard from the other four armed forces. These men and women, despite the hardships, are the reason the stations and SAR in the U.S. Coast Guard work. But again, who are these men and women and why do they continue to risk their lives for others with very little in return? Due to the apparently strong desire by the leadership of the service to keep anonymous the men and women who fill the ranks of the U.S. Coast Guard, this question is difficult to answer. In examining the few books available on the people who work in search and rescue, and of the rescues themselves, we catch glimpses of the lifesavers.

Perhaps the best description of why people in the U.S. Life-Saving Service pushed out into gale-swept seas using human muscle against the fury of the sea comes from the written investigations undertaken by U.S. Revenue Cutter Service officers. The officers served tours of duty as inspectors of the Life-Saving Service stations. Part of their duty was to investigate wrecks within their area of operations. Many inspectors remarked on the "brave and persistent efforts" and wrote of "prodigies of heroism" and "unflinching heroism." The rescues in this book also show a resourcefulness and a willingness to improvise to accomplish their mission.

As one writing in the twenty-first century, and without sufficient documentation, it is not only difficult but also presumptuous to speak for lifesavers of the U.S. Life-Saving Service era. Judging by the skimpy records, however, it appears these men never looked upon themselves as heroes. Rather, they saw themselves as watermen who grew up around the sea and did their best to help those in distress upon the water.

If the information on who crewed the stations of the U.S. Life-Saving Service is skimpy, then the information on those serving in the U.S. Coast Guard is almost nonexistent. Since the founding of the service in 1915, there have been only two books and one autobiography published concerning those serving at stations.[8] The rescues in this book show that the men and women at the modern U.S. Coast Guard stations carry all the traits of their predecessors, that is, they are brave, have a sense of duty, and are resourceful. Like their predecessors, they struggle with low pay and long hours of duty. Unlike their predecessors, they must cope with a disconnected leadership at the headquarters level and a feeling of being forgotten.

No one interviewed for this book ever looked upon their rescues as heroic. Paul Dupuis, who, along with his crew, rescued people from a blazing barge filled with fireworks, said his crew did "exactly what 99.9 percent of [U.S. Coast Guard crews] do[:] 'Get it done.'"[9] Chief Warrant Officer F. Scott Clendenin said that anyone responding to a call of distress during heavy weather conditions in a small motor lifeboat, "when all your senses are screaming not to go, is a hero."[10] Boatswain's Mate 1st Class Bernard C. Webber, for example, knew what awaited him in that gale-swept February night of 1952. Yet he and his crew left the shelter of the harbor. Literally thousands of men and women of the U.S. Coast Guard's small boat stations have set out when all their "senses are screaming not to go." Some have received recognition for what they accomplished; most have not.

The question remains: Why do people willingly push out into a raging sea? Again, an outsider feels trying to articulate the reasons is presumptuous. As one senior chief petty officer remarked, "Until you've been on a motor lifeboat in heavy seas and have watched as the bow plunges downward in steep swells, and your stomach is tied up in knots because you are not certain you are going to come up again, and all the time the crew is relaxed because the chief is on the wheel, then you don't know what you are talking about."[11] Headquarters no doubt would point out training allows people to have the confidence to push out into heavy seas. To some extent this is correct. Others might point out that some people are "adrenalin junkies." The sound of the SAR alarm ringing throughout a station can put a jolt of adrenalin into a person's system that is indescribable. Many live for this. Someone once remarked, "Risk is extra life."

Lt. Michael F. White, at one time the commanding officer of Station Cape Disappointment, wrote an explanation for the willingness of crews to put out into heavy seas. White felt that people at the small boat stations have a sense of "a willingness to act, even at extreme risk . . . particularly when lives are at stake."[12]

There is one factor that makes a cadre of people willing to push out into heavy seas, at great risk to their own lives, and to bear up under policies dictated upon them by a disconnected headquarters, and that is the saving of lives. Many crewmembers tried to describe how it felt to save a life. While most could not find adequate words, there was no doubt that the experience was nearly religious, comparable to Saul's experience on the road to Damascus. Cdr. Michael C. Monteith, a former commanding officer of Station Cape Disappointment, said about saving a life, "It's a rare moment that, when it's all over, you reflect on just how precious, temporal, and delicate life is. It humbles you, not vice versa. I'm one of the very few officers in the U.S. Coast Guard who has actually reached over the gunwale of a small boat and pulled a person from the sea; and if I could have only one memory in life to cherish, I think that would be it."[13]

After the rescue of *Ephraim Williams* in December 1885 by Keeper Benjamin Daily's crew, a U.S. Revenue Cutter Service officer wrote in his report, "These poor, plain men, dwellers upon the lonely sands of Hatteras, took their lives in their hands, and, at the most imminent risk, crossed the most tumultuous sea . . . , and all for what? That others might live to see home and friends."[14] The stories in this book reflect the heroic deeds of many men and women who have experienced the feelings of rescuing someone from the sea. Some also have felt the anguish of watching people die, despite their best efforts. To date, there has been no Homer, Herman Melville, or Charles Dana to record their deeds so that Americans recognize they have always had maritime heroes living among them. Until that time, if you wish to see ordinary men and women who perform heroic deeds, visit a U.S. Coast Guard small boat rescue station.

Notes

Publishers have given permission to use material from the following Dennis L. Noble works: Portions of chapter 1 appeared in a different form in *That Others Might Live: The U.S. Life-Saving Service, 1878–1914* (Annapolis: Naval Institute Press, 1994). Portions of chapter 4 appeared in a different form in *That Others Might Live: The U.S. Life-Saving Service, 1878–1914* (Annapolis: Naval Institute Press, 1994) and "Lawrence O. Lawson: An Extraordinary Keeper," *Wreck & Rescue: The Journal of the U.S. Life-Saving Service Heritage Association* 6, no. 1 (May 2003): 14–16. Portions of chapter 12 appeared in a different form in *Lifeboat Sailors: Disasters, Rescues, and the Perilous Future of the Coast Guard's Small Boat Stations* (Washington, D.C.: Brassey's, 2000) and "End of an Era," *Wreck & Rescue: The Journal of the U.S. Life-Saving Service Heritage Association* 15 (Fall 2000): 15–18. Portions of chapter 13 appeared in a different form in *Lifeboat Sailors: Disasters, Rescues, and the Perilous Future of the Coast Guard's Small Boat Stations* (Washington, D.C.: Brassey's, 2000) and "Lifesaver," *Wreck & Rescue: The Journal of the U.S. Life-Saving Service Heritage Association* 4, no. 4 (Fall 2000): 8–11. Portions of chapter 14 appeared in a different form in *The Rescue of the Gale Runner: Death, Heroism, and the U.S. Coast Guard* (Gainesville: University Press of Florida, 2002).

Chapter 1. Brave and Persistent Efforts

1. Bennett, *Surfboats, Rockets, and Carronades,* 14–16; Noble and O'Brien, *That Others Might Live,* 5.
2. Noble and O'Brien, *That Others Might Live,* 5.
3. For material on the Massachusetts Humane Society, see Howe, *Humane Society of the Commonwealth of Massachusetts.*
4. Noble, *Legacy,* 4.
5. U.S. Life-Saving Service, *Annual Report of the Operations of the United States Life-Saving Service . . . 1876* (hereafter cited as *ARUSLSS,* followed by appropriate year), 76.
6. Davis, "Life Saving Stations," 310.
7. Quoted in Means, "Heavy Sea Running," 226; *ARUSLSS,* 1876, 76.
8. Senate Committee on Commerce, *Letter from the Secretary of the Treasury Communicating . . the Present Condition of the Life-Saving Stations on the Coasts of New Jersey and Long Island,* 42d Cong., 2d sess., 1872; "Synopsis of Report of Capt. John Faunce on Inspection of Life-Saving Stations on Coasts of Long Island and New Jersey, August 1871," "Summary of Expenditures Required for New and Old Life-Saving Stations. Coasts of Long Island and Jersey, September 1871," and "Estimate for Coast of New Jersey, October 12, 1871, John Faunce, Captain and Inspector," all in "Miscellaneous, 1849–75," Box 1, Records of the U.S. Coast Guard, RG 26, NARA (hereafter cited as RUSCG).
9. Noble, *That Others Might Live,* 32.
10. Noble, *Legacy,* 9.
11. Ibid.
12. Ibid, 11.
13. Davis, "Life Saving Stations," 310.
14. Kimball, *Organization and Methods,* 10.
15. Unless otherwise noted, all material on the wreck and rescue of the Taulane is from *ARUSLSS,* 1880, 106–20; O'Connor, *Heroes of the Storm,* 81–92; Noble, *That Others Might Live,* 1–5.
16. Unless otherwise noted, all material on the work of the Cleveland Station comes from *Journal, U.S. Life-Saving Station, Cleveland, Ohio, April 20, 1883 to April 12, 1884,* Federal Records Center, Suitland, Md.; *ARUSLSS,* 1891, 130–31, 133, 145–47.

17. The official report of the rescue of the *Sophia Minch* does not record the first names of Customs Inspector Bates or Pryor, Duffy, and Tovat. *ARUSLSS,* 1891, 130–31, 133, 145–47.

18. For material on Frederick T. Hatch's work and rescue as a lighthouse keeper, see Oleszewski, *Lighthouse Adventures,* 186–95.

19. Unless otherwise noted, all material on the wreck and rescue of the *San Albano* is from *ARUSLSS,* 1892, 35–39.

Chapter 2. Unflinching Heroism

1. Noble, *That Others Might Live,* 85–90.

2. Ibid., 94–98, 101–3.

3. Unless otherwise noted, all material on the wreck and rescue of the *Ephraim Williams* is from *ARUSLSS,* 1885, 162–64. A very good secondary source is Stick, *Graveyard of the Atlantic,* 112–15.

4. Material on the wreck and rescue of the *Rawson* is found in *ARUSLSS,* 1905, 38–40, 136.

5. Material on the wreck and rescue of the *Margaret* is found in *ARUSLSS,* 1913, 62–66.

Chapter 3. Prodigies of Heroism

1. Quoted in Noble, *That Others Might Live,* 130.

2. *ARUSLSS,* 1899, 233–40.

3. Unless otherwise noted, all material on the wreck and rescue of the *Dyer* is from *ARUSLSS,* 1889, 27–29.

4. The Jerry's Point Station was a new one, built on Great Island in Portsmouth Harbor in 1887. The property was under the War Department, and it was reclaimed in 1907. The station eventually was rebuilt on Wood Island, Maine. Shanks, York, and Shanks, *U.S. Life-Saving Service,* 27.

5. Journal, Gull Shoal Station, North Carolina, 18 August 1899, Federal Records Center, Suitland, Md. Unless otherwise noted, all material on Midgett's rescue is found in *ARUSLSS,* 1900, 25–28; Scrapbooks of the U.S. Life-Saving Service, 1899–1900, RUSCG (hereafter cited as Scrapbooks, followed by date); Stick, *Graveyard of the Atlantic,* 166–68.

6. Unless otherwise noted, all material on the wreck and rescue of the *Abbott* is from *ARUSLSS,* 1903, 26–28, 133.

7. Bertholf would become the last captain commandant of the U.S. Revenue Cutter Service and the first captain commandant of the new U.S. Coast Guard. For a biography of Bertholf, see Kroll, *Commodore Ellsworth P. Bertholf.*

Chapter 4. Angels in Oilskins

1. Noble, *That Others Might Live,* 60–61.
2. Quoted in Noble, *Legacy,* 15–16.
3. In over twenty years of research on maritime rescue by the U.S. Coast Guard, I have seen or heard of only three diaries.
4. Material on Lawson appeared in different form in Noble, "Lawrence O. Lawson," 14–16. All material on Keeper Lawrence O. Lawson, unless otherwise noted, comes from photocopied material sent to the author from the Evanston Historical Society, Evanston, Illinois.
5. Scrapbooks, 1900.
6. All material on the *Calumet* rescue, except the direct quotes from the Evanston Historical Society material, are from *ARUSLSS,* 1890, 223.
7. Material on Roberge obtained from a family scrapbooks and interviews with his son, Capt. T. L. Roberge, U.S. Coast Guard (Ret.) in 1993 at his home in Port Angeles, Washington. Captain Roberge has since died.
8. Roberge married the daughter of the keeper of the Cape Disappointment Light Station and thus had some type of contact with three of the five organizations that would eventually make up the U. S. Coast Guard: the U. S. Revenue Cutter Service, the U. S. Life-Saving Service and the U. S. Lighthouse Service. U.S. Coast Guard, *Register of the Commissioned and Warrant Officers,* 1962 (hereafter cited as *Register,* followed by date), 116.
9. Dalton, *Life Savers of Cape Cod,* 70–72.
10. Scrapbooks; "The Life-Saving Station," photocopy from unknown source in Historian of the U.S. Coast Guard Files, Washington, D.C. (hereafter cited as Historian Files).
11. All material on Morgan's work is found in Edith Morgan File, Historian Files.
12. All material on Griesser's work is found in *ARUSLSS,* 1901, 41–42, 103–4. The official record of the U.S. Life-Saving Service's account of the rescue records only "W. W. Griesser."

13. The wreck and rescue of the *Noyes* is found in *ARUSLSS*, 1903, 127–28.

Chapter 5. March 1902

1. Galluzzo, "Big Shoes to Fill," 4.
2. Unless otherwise noted, material on the deaths of the Monomoy crew is found in *ARUSLSS*, 1902, 32–36.
3. Galluzzo, "Big Shoes to Fill," 4.
4. The *Annual Report* states this was "Francisco Bloomer, a skilled surfman," while Galluzzo states it was Surfman Walter C. Bloomer. *ARUSLSS*, 1902, 35; Galluzzo, "Big Shoes to Fill," 4.
5. Kimball, *Joshua James*, 100.
6. Ibid., 16–17.
7. Ibid., 74.
8. Baarslag, *Coast Guard to the Rescue*, 74.
9. Ibid.
10. Ibid.
11. Ibid., 74–75.
12. Ibid., 76.
13. Ibid., 77.
14. Ibid.
15. Ibid., 77–78.
16. Ibid., 79.
17. Quoted in Kimball, *Joshua James*, 95.

Chapter 6. New Weapons against the Sea

1. Holland, *America's Lighthouses*, 32.
2. Ibid., 32, 37.
3. *ARUSLSS*, 1910, 17.
4. Bennett, "Life-Savers," 63.
5. Evans, *United States Coast Guard*, 206–7.
6. Evans's *United States Coast Guard* and Johnson's *Guardians of the Sea* remain the best works on the evolution of the U.S. Coast Guard. All material on the merging of the U.S. Life-Saving Service and U.S. Revenue Cutter Service is found in *Economy and Efficiency in the*

Government Service: Message of the President of the United States Transmitting Reports on the Commission on Economy and Efficiency, 62d Cong., 2d sess., H. Doc. 670, 4 April 1912, 378–89, 389–97. Evans, *United States Coast Guard,* 215.

7. See Noble, "Unless There Was a Death," for a discussion of these issues.

8. I am indebted to William D. Wilkinson, the internationally recognized expert on U.S. Coast Guard rescue craft, for material he sent on the 36-foot motor lifeboat. "U.S. Coast Guard Motor Lifeboats, 1918–1956," in author's files.

9. Within the U.S. Coast Guard's small boat community, there is a belief that the 52-foot motor lifeboats were designed specifically for the Pacific Northwest. Scheina, in his work on cutters and craft of the U.S. Coast Guard during World War II, shows that one of the two wooden 52-foot motor lifeboats was stationed at Sandy Hook, New Jersey. When the U.S. Coast Guard built steel 52-footers, however, all have been stationed in the Pacific Northwest. Scheina, *Cutters and Craft of World War II,* 251; Scheina, *Cutters and Craft, 1946–1990,* 194.

10. Scheina, *Cutters and Craft, 1946–1990,* 190–96, 203–6.

11. Johnson, *Guardians,* 42; Kroll, *Ellsworth P. Bertholf,* 118; Scheina, *Coast Guard Aviation,* 10.

12. Charles E. Sugden, born 6 September 1883, at Stockbridge, Massachusetts, graduated from the U.S. Revenue Cutter Service's School of Instruction on 11 March 1909 as a third lieutenant. He was one of the first two U.S. Coast Guard officers assigned to flight training at the U.S. Naval Air Station Pensacola, Florida, where he became U.S. Coast Guard aviator number 4 and U.S. Naval Aviator number 43. Sugden retired as a captain on 1 August 1946. For his work at Ile Tudy, he was, according to his official biography, authorized "to accept, if awarded, the rank of 'Chevalier of the Legion of Honor of France' for his service overseas. Owing to some later oversight that award was never fully authorized. He, however, received the Victory Medal and a silver star for his campaign ribbon for meritorious services rendered . . . during the war." Captain Charles E. Sugden File, Historian Files.

13. Scheina, *Coast Guard Aviation,* 13–14.

14. Ibid., 14–15.

15. Ibid., 16, 19.

16. "ARCTURUS; rescue by; damage resultant," RUSCG (hereafter cited as ARCTURUS; Von Paulsen's official report on the incident.) Carl C. Von Paulsen was born in Helena, Montana, 24 January 1891. He graduated from the U.S. Revenue Cutter Service's School of Instruction as a third lieutenant on 7 June 1913. He graduated from the Naval Air Training School, Pensacola, Florida, in June 1920, as U.S. Coast Guard Aviator number 6 on 6 December 1920. He also graduated from the U.S. Army's Primary Flying School in June 1922 and graduated with honors from the U.S. Army Advanced Bombardment Flying School, Kelly Field, San Antonio, Texas, on 17 December 1922. Von Paulsen retired as a captain on 1 June 1945. Captain Carl C. Von Paulsen, USCG File, Historian Files.

17. Baarslag, *Coast Guard to the Rescue,* 12.

18. ARCTURUS.

19. Baarslag, *Coast Guard to the Rescue,* 14.

20. ARCTURUS; Baarslag, *Coast Guard to the Rescue,* 15.

21. ARCTURUS; Baarslag, *Coast Guard to the Rescue,* 17.

22. President Franklin D. Roosevelt had transferred the U.S. Coast Guard to the Navy on 1 November 1941; Johnson, *Guardians,* 195.

23. Quoted in Beard, *Wonderful Flying Machines,* 2.

24. Ibid., 2.

25. Scheina, *History of Coast Guard Aviation,* 25; Barrett Thomas Beard to author, e-mail, 28 December 2002.

26. Waters, "Finally the Twain Did Meet," 99.

27. Ibid., 98.

28. Scheina, *Coast Guard Aviation,* 25.

29. Beard, *Wonderful Flying Machines,* 46, 48, 55, 58, 59–60, 66, 70, 78–79, 82–83, 90, 118, 123, 124–25.

30. Quoted in ibid., 49. All material on the first humanitarian mission flown by Erickson, unless otherwise noted, is in ibid., 49–50.

31. All material on the Labrador rescue, unless otherwise noted, is in Beard, *Wonderful Flying Machines,* 98–102; Nalty, Noble, and Strobridge, *Wrecks, Rescues and Investigations,* 294.

32. Beard, *Wonderful Flying Machines,* 108–9. At a gathering of enlisted aviation retirees at Port Angeles, Washington, on 20 October 2001, I heard many stories about MacDiarmid. I gained most of my material

from ADCS Jack Halsey, U.S. Coast Guard (Ret.) (hereafter cited as Interview).

33. Interview.
34. Waters, "Finally the Twain Did Meet," 92
35. Beard, *Wonderful Flying Machines,* 109.
36. Waters, *Rescue at Sea,* 104.
37. Ibid., 104–5.
38. Ibid., 105.
39. Scheina, *Coast Guard Aviation,* 31–32.
40. Waters, "Finally the Twain Did Meet," 98.
41. Quoted in Beard, *Wonderful Flying Machines,* 116.
42. Ibid.
43. Ibid.
44. Ibid.
45. Quoted in ibid., 117.

Chapter 7. Business as Usual

1. Unless otherwise noted, all material on the rescue of the men from the barge is contained within "Wreck Report, August 6, 1918," RUSCG.
2. Barnett, "Lifesaving Guns," 9.
3. Ibid.
4. Ibid.
5. Stick, *Graveyard of the Atlantic,* 204.
6. Lester, "When You're Raised Around the Water," 6.
7. John Allen Midgett enlisted in the U.S. Life-Saving Service in 1890 and was named keeper of the Chicamacomico Station on June 1916. John Allen Midgett File, Historian Files; Bearss, "'Mirlo' Rescue," 385 n. 5. Bearss's article contains the best documented source of the *Mirlo* rescue, and I drew heavily upon it.
8. Bearss, "'Mirlo' Rescue," 389.
9. Ibid., 387, 389. Despite extensive research, Bearss was not able to obtain the first name or initials of Droscher.
10. Stick claims the *Mirlo* struck mines, *Graveyard of the Atlantic,* 204, but Bearss's evidence is convincing that the sinking was by *U-117*. See Bearss, "'Mirlo' Rescue," 387 n.12.

11. Quoted in Bearss, "'Mirlo' Rescue," 392.

12. Ibid.

13. Ibid., 385, 392.

14. All descriptions of the lifesavers are from ibid., 385 n. 6, 390 n. 17, 398 n. 36.

15. Ibid., 393; Stick, *Graveyard of the Atlantic,* 205–6.

16. Bearss, "'Mirlo' Rescue," 393.

17. Ibid., 393–94; Stick, *Graveyard of the Atlantic,* 206.

18. Bearss, "'Mirlo' Rescue," 394.

19. Stick, *Graveyard of the Atlantic,* 207.

20. Bearss, "'Mirlo' Rescue," 395.

21. Ibid.

22. Ibid.

23. Quoted in ibid., 395–96.

24. Ibid., 398; Stick, *Graveyard of the Atlantic,* 207.

25. Kaplan and Hunt, *This Is the Coast Guard,* 278.

26. Ibid.

27. Noble and O'Brien, *Sentinels,* 40; Stonehouse, "Gold Medal Shipwreck," 4.

28. Noble and O'Brien, *Sentinels,* 40.

29. Ibid., 40–41.

30. Stonehouse, "Gold Medal Shipwreck," 4

31. Ibid.

32. Ibid. The SC-438 was renamed twice—*Cook* and *Island*—and during World War II, it served as the cutter *Bonneville.* It was decommissioned on 22 September 1945. Scheina, *Cutters and Craft of World War II,* 200–201.

33. Noble and O'Brien, *Sentinels,* 41–42; Stonehouse, "Gold Medal Shipwreck," 4.

34. Stonehouse, "Gold Medal Shipwreck," 5.

35. Noble and O'Brien, *Sentinels,* 42.

36. Stonehouse, "Gold Medal Shipwreck," 6.

37. Noble and O'Brien, *Sentinels,* 42.

38. Stonehouse, "Gold Medal Shipwreck," 6.

39. Wolff, "One Hundred Years of Rescue," 33.

40. *ARUSLSS,* 1876, 11–14.

41. Untitled and undated newspaper clipping located in the files of the Pictured Rocks National Lakeshore, Munising, Michigan.

42. Ibid.

43. Noble and O'Brien, *Sentinels,* 42.

44. Ibid., 43, 45.

45. Ibid., 42.

46. Stonehouse, "Gold Medal Shipwreck," 7.

47. Ibid. Photocopy of a photocopy of the log book of the Grand Marais Station in the possession of Frederick Stonehouse.

48. Ibid.

49. The Historian of the U.S. Coast Guard's web site lists the following as receiving the Gold Life Saving Medal: John O. Anderson, Alfred E. Kristofferson, Leon E. Alford, George Olsen (Stonehouse has the name as Olson), Glen Wells, Edward J. Spencer, Russell Martin, William Campbell, Joseph G. McShea. There is some question as to the names of the civilians who helped in the rescue. Stonehouse has the names as Ambose and Joseph Graham, Ora Endress, and James MacDonald. Frederick Stonehouse to author, e-mails, 3 and 4 December 2003.

50. Galluzzo, "Those Guys Got Plenty of Guts," 14.

51. Ibid.

52. Some Coast Guard Rescues and Incidents, Acc. 87-3-18/7 (hereafter cited as Memoirs). In 1909, Hilman married Eliza Jane Armstrong, a member of one of the early families of the area. They had three children; two lived to adulthood.

53. Galluzzo, "Those Guys Got Plenty of Guts," 14; Memoirs of Fridolph Persson, p. 1.

54. Galluzzo, "Those Guys Got Plenty of Guts," 15–16; Trinidad File, Columbia River Maritime Museum (hereafter cited as Trinidad File). This file consists of photocopied newspaper clippings concerning the *Trinidad* case.

55. Gibbs, *Pacific Graveyard,* 152.

56. Galluzzo, "Those Guys Got Plenty of Guts," 15–16; Trinidad File.

57. Ibid.

58. Memoirs, 8.

59. Galluzzo, "Those Guys Got Plenty of Guts," 16.

60. Memoirs, 9; Trinidad File.

61. Ibid.

62. Ibid.

63. Ibid.

64. Ibid., 9–10.

65. Ibid., 9.

66. Galluzzo, "Those Guys Got Plenty of Guts," 17.

67. Trinidad File.

68. Memoirs, 10.

69. Trinidad File.

70. Memoirs.

71. Ibid; Trinidad File.

72. All material on the *Emidio* case, unless otherwise noted, comes from the scrapbook of the Humboldt Bay U.S. Coast Guard Station, Samoa, California (hereafter cited as Humboldt Scrapbooks). The material consists of photocopies of the following: Senior Coast Guard Officer, Twelfth Naval District, 30 December 1941 to Chief Boatswain (L) Garner J. Churchill; "Sinking of the EMIDIO," by Melvin A. Krei, typescript, n.d.; U.S. Coast Guard, Deeds of Valor from the Annals of the U. S. Coast Guard (Washington, D.C.: GPO, 1943), 16–20; obituary from unknown newspaper. I am indebted to CWO Richard K. Loster, Surface Operations Officer, Group Humboldt Bay, California, for providing me the photocopies and for other assistance on the *Emidio* case and on Garner J. Churchill. The Blunt's Reef Lightship at this time was anchored at 40-26.1 North and 124-30.3 West, "about 4.55 [miles and] 266 [degrees] from Cape Mendocino Light. Served as a reference mark for coastwise traffic in passing clear of Blunt's Reef and other shoal spots in the vicinity." Flint, *Lightships of the United States Government*, n.p.

73. Churchill's promotion to warrant officer is recorded in *Register,* 1940, 83. Information on the rescue of the *Reta* is in Noble, *Southwest Pacific*, 10.

74. Ralph C. Shanks Jr. and Janetta Thompson Shanks claim that the U.S. Navy commander of the naval radio station refused to let Churchill cross the bar. "Finally, Chief Churchill could stand it no longer. He telephoned the Navy commander informing him that the Coast Guard was going to the rescue." Shanks and Shanks, *Lighthouses and Lifeboats*, 188–89.

75. Van Dorn, *Oceanography and Seamanship*, 187.

76. After the weather moderated, the cutter Shawnee took the survivors of the *Emidio* off the lightship. Shanks and Shanks, *Lighthouses and Lifeboats*, 191.

77. After being declared a menace to navigation, the stern was sunk.

78. Churchill received the Silver Life Saving Medal, two unit citations, four area citations, and thirty-two letters of commendation. He retired in 1955 as a lieutenant commander with thirty-one years of service. Garner J. Churchill died, at the age of eighty-three, on 28 December 1983. Humboldt Scrapbook.

79. U.S. Coast Guard, *U.S. Coast Guard at War* 14:34.

80. Ibid.; Noble, "Soviets on a Shoestring," 141.

81. Noble, "Soviets on a Shoestring," 141; completed questionnaire from Mike James to author, 1989, in author's files (hereafter cited as James questionnaire).

82. Noble, "Soviets on a Shoestring," 141.

83. The rescue of the Lamut's crew has been used by the service over the years to show the improvisation of U.S. Coast Guard crews. The use of shoestrings has always been the centerpiece of the rescue. Recently, some have questioned whether the crew used shoelaces or bandages. The caption of the photographs taken at the time of the rescue states shoelaces were used. Caption on the back of photograph of Lamut rescue, photographic files, Historian Files. The reprinted War Diary of 10 April 1943 reports bandages were used; Nalty, Noble, and Strobridge, *Wrecks, Rescues, and Investigations*, 152; Noble, "Soviets on a Shoestring," 141.

84. Quoted in Noble, "Soviets on a Shoestring," 141.

85. Nalty, Noble, and Strobridge, *Wrecks, Rescues, and Investigations*, 152.

86. Ibid.

87. James questionnaire.

Chapter 8. The Rescue of *Pendelton*

1. The cutters involved were *Yakutat* (WAVP-380), *McCulloch* (WAVP-386), *Eastwind* (WAGB-279), and *Acushnet* (WAT-167). A "Gruman Amphibian from Quonset Point, R.I." also assisted. Earle, "Saga of Ships," 12–13, 16–18. Johnson mentions that *Unimak* (WAVP- 379)

also participated, while Earle has no mention of the cutter. Johnson, *Guardians,* 287.

2. Information on the *Pendelton* is from "Marine Board of Investigation; Structural Failure of tanker PENDELTON," Historian of the U.S. Coast Guard.

3. Ibid.

4. Webster, *"Pendelton* Rescue," 66.

5. *Fort Mercer* was a 10,266-ton 503-foot T-2 type tanker. "Marine Board of Investigation; Structural Failure of tanker FORT MERCER," Historian of the U.S. Coast Guard; Webber, *Chatham,* 43. Frump, *Until the Sea Shall Free Them,* discusses the problems of T-2 tankers.

6. Unless otherwise noted, all quotations are from Webber, *Chatham,* 43–52.

7. Ibid. There was also another 36-footer from the Brant Point Station, on Nantucket Island, sent out on this night. Earle, "Saga of Ships," 15, 16.

8. McCulloch and the other motor lifeboat from Chatham "saw to the bow of the *Pendelton.* . . . One man [from *Pendelton*] jumped into the turbulent sea . . . , but could not be located." No one on the bow section survived. Johnson, *Guardians,* 288. *Yakutat* took off four survivors from the *Fort Mercer*'s bow. *Eastwind* took off three sailors from the stern of *Fort Mercer,* while *Acushnet* took off eighteen from the tanker's stern. At least thirteen sailors elected to remain aboard the stern. Johnson feels that the survivors on the stern of *Fort Mercer* "might have survived without Coast Guard assistance." Johnson puts the total number of sailors rescued at seventy-one, while Earle puts the number at seventy. Johnson, *Guardians,* 288; Earle, "Saga of Ships," 12.

9. Ibid., 46. Webber was born 9 May 1928 and entered the Merchant Marine at the age of sixteen. He enlisted in the U.S. Coast Guard on 26 February 1946, with the following assignments: Highland Light Station, Gay Head Light and Lifeboat Station, cutter *Dexter* (WHEC-85), Monomoy Lookout Station, Chatham Loran Monitoring Station, Chatham Lifeboat Station, a patrol boat, WPB-CG-83388, Nauset Lifeboat Station, Race Point Lifeboat Station. All these assignments were in Massachusetts. Then to the tug (WYT 64301) at Southwest Harbor, Maine. He returned to Massachusetts again aboard the Nantucket/Relief Lightship (WAL 534), then back to Chatham Lifeboat Station to the Cross Rip Lightship (WAL 525) to the buoy tender *White Sage* (WLM 544) to the *Point Banks* (WPB

82327), all in Massachusetts. Webber, while aboard the *Point Banks,* was sent to Vietnam and returned to the United States for assignment aboard the buoy tender *Hornbeam* (WLB 394) in Massachusetts. He retired on 1 September 1966 while serving in *Hornbeam* as warrant officer 1. Webber now resides in the southeastern United States. Bernard C. Webber to author, e-mail, 23 January 2003.

10. Webster, *"Pendelton* Rescue," 67.

11. Completed questionnaire from Ervin E. Maske to author, 25 April 2003 (hereafter cited as Maske questionnaire). Maske was born 24 April 1929 at Marinette, Wisconsin. He entered the U.S. Coast Guard at Green Bay, Wisconsin, in 1950 "because my older brother was in the Coast Guard." He left the U.S. Coast Guard at the end of his first enlistment and returned to Marinette, Wisconsin. Ervin E. Maske "died suddenly" of a "massive heart attack" in October 2003. Anita B. Jevne, daughter of Maske, to author, e-mail, 28 October 2003.

12. Webber, *Chatham,* 47–48. Johnson and Earle state Webber was guided to the *Pendelton* by a radar operator at Chatham. Webber denies this in his book and denies it in a recent e-mail. Further, Johnson and Earle write that U.S. Coast Guard aircraft helped illuminate the scene, which is not shown in Webber's account, nor in a latter e-mail. Johnson, *Guardians,* 287–88; Earle, "Saga of Ships," 15, 18; Webber to author, e-mail, 23 January 2003.

13. Webber, *Chatham,* 48–49.

14. Maske questionnaire.

15. Webber, *Chatham,* 50. "Then all hell broke loose on the radio[,] every cutter within earshot had orders for me, wanting me to deliver my cargo out to them no matter where they were. I said to myself phooey, no way. I was tired just beat, frozen and in no mood to play games . . . and concentrated on getting my cargo to safety. From then on the whole deal took on a political posture, there was talk I should be court-martialed." Bernard C. Webber to author, e-mail, 23 January 2003.

16. Completed questionnaire from Richard P. Livesey to author, 9 March 2003, in author's files. Livesey was born on 21 February 1930 and enlisted in the U.S. Coast Guard at Lowell, Massachusetts, on 31 March 1947. He retired on 31 October 1967 as a BM1. Livesey now resides in the southeastern United States.

17. Webber, *Chatham,* 50–51.

18. A total of five Gold Life Saving Medals were awarded for the work in the *Fort Mercer* and *Pendelton* rescues: four to Webber and his crew and one to Ens. William R. Kiely of the *Yakutat*. Silver Life Saving Medals were awarded to Ens. Gilbert E. Carmichael, Engineman 2d Class Paul R. Black, Seaman Webster G. Terwilliger, and Seaman Apprentice Edward A. Mason Jr., all from the *Yakutat*. The high awards to the *Yakutat* crewmen were for their efforts in a boat between *Yakutat* and *Fort Mercer*. Earle, "Saga of Ships," 16.

    Even though the rescue of the *Pendelton* is one of the icons of the U.S. Coast Guard, Webber told me, "You are the first person writing a book that has directly come to me for any information I have." Webber to author, e-mail, 23 January 2003.

19. Webber to author, 23 January 2003.

20. Livesey's comments on Myers are in his completed questionnaire.

21. Webber to author, e-mail, 23 January 2003.

Chapter 9. I Thought It Was the End

1. David Pearson, Curator, Columbia River Maritime Museum, to author, e-mail, 2 April 2003.

2. Viola and Margolis, *Magnificent Voyagers*, 20, 150, 268.

3. Unless otherwise noted, all material on the *Mermaid* case, including the description of the area at the mouth of the Columbia River, is in U.S. Coast Guard Board of Investigation, Serial A25/5097, 14 February 1961, Seattle, Washington (hereafter cited as Board).

4. When asked why Point Adams, which is farther from the bar than Cape Disappointment, had the larger 52-foot motor lifeboat, BMCS Darrell J. Murray, U.S. Coast Guard (Ret.) replied that it was because of "politics." Because of the influence of Senator Mark Hatfield, the boat was stationed in Oregon. Darrell J. Murray, interview with author, 16 April 2003, Sequim, Washington, notes in author's files (hereafter cited as Murray interview).

5. The *Mermaid*, official number 238079, twelve gross tons and eight net tons, 34.3 by 10.7 by 5.4 feet, built of wood in 1938 at Tacoma, Washington, powered by a thirty-horsepower diesel engine, hull painted white, owned and operated by Bert E. Bergman, Chinook, Washington; Board. Times given are from the official investigation. Murray, however, recalls that the call from *Mermaid* "came in at 4:08 P.M., was logged as 4:10 p.m., with [40-footer] departing at 4:15 P.M."

Murray to author, 27 November 2003 (hereafter cited as Murray letter).

6. Darrell J. Murray enlisted in the U.S. Coast Guard Reserves on 15 May 1952. He entered onto active duty on 19 August 1955. Duty stations included a lightship; Training Center, Groton, Connecticut; Base Seattle, Washington; Lifeboat Stations Neah Bay, Washington, and Cape Disappointment, Washington; cutter *Yocona* (WAT-168), Light Station Point Wilson, Washington; cutter *Cape Henlopen* (CG-95328), Training Center Alameda, California; cutter *Boutwell* (WHEC-719); Base Boston, Massachusetts; cutter *White Bush* (WAGL-542); and Base Tongue Point, Oregon. Murray retired as a senior chief boatswain's mate on 1 January 1977. Murray letter.

7. Murray has amassed what amounts to the largest collection of material concerning the *Mermaid* case (hereafter cited as Murray collection). He has placed a portion of this in a self-published scrapbook, "First Reunion on 30th Anniversary Triumph–F/V *Mermaid* Incident." Murray shared much of his material and his memories of the incident during an extended interview.

8. Ibid.

9. Ibid. "Location of *Mermaid* was first observed in the middle of the Surf Line just North of Seaview[, Washington] Beach Approach. Surf lines as remembered were seven to nine [feet] at the time."

10. Ibid.

11. Ibid.

12. Ibid.

13. Ibid.

14. Gordon Huggins enlisted in the U.S. Coast Guard in October 1956. Duty stations included Light Station Destruction Island, Washington; Port Security Unit, Portland, Oregon; Lifeboat Station Point Adams, Oregon; Light Station Eldred Rock, Alaska; cutter *Point Marone* (CG-82331); duty in Vietnam from May 1965 to April 1966; and Depot Vancouver, Washington. Huggins left the U.S. Coast Guard in October 1966. Huggins to author, undated (hereafter cited as Huggins letter).

15. Huggins letter.

16. Murray collection.

17. Ibid.

18. Ibid.

19. Lt. Richard J. Burke Jr., commanding officer, Station Cape Disappointment to author, e-mail, 12–13 October 2003: "All surf boats [at Cape Disappointment] now carry pre-made bridles. In addition to the wire bridles used on the largest of the fishing vessels we tow in, we also carry kevlar bridles which are more expensive but last longer that the old double braded nylon bridles [and] . . . we carry 2 drogues on each surf boat. One for smaller vessels and one for larger commercial vessels."

20. "Reunion Members Reminisce," photocopy of article in files of Columbia River Maritime Museum, Astoria, Oregon.

21. Motor lifeboat crews in the Pacific Northwest have had, and continue to have, a great affection and reliance on the 52-footers. (Today they are metal.) Even though the boats are not designed to come back from a capsizing, many in the 1961 Cape Disappointment crew obviously thought they were like the 36-foot motor lifeboat. Newspapers in the region also had this mistaken impression. One headline read "Sea Tragedy Disproves Unsinkable, Non-Capsizable Boat." Murray collection.

22. "Reunion Members Reminisce." Huggins remembered the seas as estimated at forty feet. Huggins letter.

23. Ibid.

24. Information on amount of deaths is found in: "Boat Force Memorial," located in U.S. Coast Guard Headquarters, Washington, D.C.

25. Capt. Williard J. Smith served as commandant of the U.S. Coast Guard from 1966 to 1970. Both Murray and Huggins have expressed to the author displeasure at some of the investigating officer's methods and comments. Both men remarked they felt Captain Smith was fair during the course of the investigation.

26. Murray collection.

27. Ibid.

Chapter 10. It Is a Rewarding Job

1. Material on the 44-foot motor lifeboat is found in Noble, *Lifeboat Sailors*, 87–88, 214–15.

2. Material on the 41-footer and 30-foot SRB is found in ibid., 216–18.

3. All material on the Ashtabula rescue is contained in an audiotape recording made by the author of crewmembers of the station in 1977, located in author's files.

4. CWO4 Paul J. Dupuis to author, e-mail, 21 April 2003.

5. Unless otherwise noted, material on rescue is from Noble, *Lifeboat Sailors*, 172–74.

6. Dupuis to author.

7. Ibid.

8. Ibid.

9. Ibid.

10. Unless otherwise noted, information on *Bainbridge Island*'s case is from photocopied material in Medals Box, Historian Files.

11. Lt. Daniel Pickles, Commanding Officer *Bainbridge Island*, to author, e-mail, 10 November 2003.

12. Unless otherwise noted, information on Duning's rescue is from photocopied material in Medals Box, Historian Files.

Chapter 11. Helicopters and Rescue Swimmers

1. Pearcy, *Coast Guard Aircraft*, 297–303.

2. Ibid., 304–7.

3. Ibid., 106–15.

4. Ibid., 62–63, 310–13.

5. The investigation into the Marine Electric case is contained within an attachment to an e-mail from Capt. David Kunkel, U.S. Coast Guard Headquarters to author, 1 July 1999. The Marine Electric case is studied in-depth in Frump, *Until the Sea Shall Free Them*.

6. Ibid.

7. ASTCM Keith R. Jensen, Helicopter Rescue Swimmer Program Manager, U.S. Coast Guard Headquarters to author, e-mail, 8 July 1999.

8. Ibid.

9. Unless otherwise noted, all material on the rescue comes from documents reproduced in Nalty, Noble, and Strobridge, *Wrecks, Rescues and Investigations*, 344–93.

10. Material on jacking rigs is found in "Marine Casualty Report: Ocean Express (Drilling Unit)," Historian of the U.S. Coast Guard.

11. Unless otherwise noted, all quotes from Vice Admiral Thorsen are from Howard B. Thorsen to author, e-mail, 26 November 2002.

12. Unless otherwise noted, material on this rescue is from Schreiner, *Mayday! Mayday!* 20–33.

13. "Rescue Swimmer's Heroics Cap 2 1/2 Years of Practice," from the *Portland Oregonian,* photocopy, n.d., n.p., Coast Guard File, Columbia River Maritime Museum, Astoria, Oregon.

14. Ibid.

15. Ibid.

16. Kelly Mogk attended Officer Candidate School and graduated as an ensign in February 1994. She went to flight school and received her wings in May 1996. In 2003, Kelly Mogk, with nineteen years of service, continued to serve in U.S. Coast Guard aviation. Interestingly, at one of her duty stations William W. Peterson, now a captain, was her commanding officer. Kelly Mogk to author, e-mail, 16 October 2003.

17. Barrett T. Beard has written the most definitive account of Odom's struggle. Beard audiotaped most of the people involved in the *Mirage* case. I have borrowed heavily from his article and all quotes are from the article. Beard, "Nineteen, Talk to Me!" 66–71.

Chapter 12. Station Yaquina Bay, Oregon

1. CWO John D. Dodd, former Commanding Officer, Yaquina Bay Station, to author, e-mail, 9 April 2003.

2. Material on McAdams appeared in a different form in Noble, *Lifeboat Sailors,* 32–48, and from McAdams, audiotaped interview with author, 17 September 1996, Yaquina Bay Station. Transcript in author's files.

3. Unless otherwise noted, material on Clendenin appeared in a different form in Noble, "End of an Era," 15–18.

4. Information on Clendenin's surf rescue is in "Rescue!" *AFRAS Newsletter: Association for Rescue at Sea* (Summer 2003): 4.

Chapter 13. Into the Twenty-first Century

1. CWO4 Kenneth D. Stuber, Commanding Officer, National Motor Lifeboat School, to author, e-mail, 3 November 2003; other material on the 47-foot motor lifeboat is found in the information sheet from Textron Marine and Land, www.systems.textron.com, and "47-foot Motor Lifeboat (MLB)," a U.S. Coast Guard data sheet, 14 March 2003, at www.uscg.mil/datasheet/47mlb.htm.

2. All material on the rescue of C. J. Hubbs appears in a different form in Noble, *Lifeboat Sailors.*

3. Unless otherwise noted, all information on the ice rescue is from Jeffery Kihlmire, audiotaped interview with author, 1996, Station Cape Disappointment, Washington. Transcript in author's files.

4. Unless otherwise noted, material on *Lee Rose* rescue comes from crewmembers, audiotaped interview with author, 12 March 1997, Station Grays Harbor. Transcript in author's files. Interviewed were Daniel C. Butenschon, Eric C. Forslund, Mike Fratusco, Brian Gaunt, Randy Lewis, Randy Merritt, and Daniel L. Smock.

5. Unless otherwise noted, all quotes by Carola are from Carola audiotaped interview with author, 26 February 2003, Yaquina Bay Station. Tape in author's files.

6. Wilder, "I'm Gonna Die!" 19.

7. Comment is also repeated in the official SAR folder for case; see UCN 85, Station Oregon Inlet, North Carolina. Case file folder obtain through a Freedom of Information Act request; Wilder, "I'm Gonna Die!" 19.

8. Wilder, "I'm Gonna Die!" 19.

9. Ibid.

10. *Miss Brittany* case appeared in a different form in Noble, "Lifesaver," 8–11. Quotes from Robert Greenfield are from *Miss Brittany* debrief, located in case folder, SAR folder, UCN 280, Station Cape Disappointment, Washington. Case folder obtained through a Freedom of Information Act request.

11. Beth Rasmussen to author, 18 December 2003.

12. Unless otherwise noted, all quotes from D'Amelio are from D'Amelio, audiotaped interview with author, 29 January 2003, Station Cape Disappointment, Washington. Tape in author's files.

13. Unless otherwise noted, all material relating to Forslund are in Forslund to author, e-mail, 14 July 2003.

14. Unless otherwise noted, all quotes and material on Slade are from Slade, audiotaped interview with author, 29 January 2003, Station Cape Disappointment, Washington. Tape in author's files. Shortly after this case, Slade received a transfer to the National Motor Lifeboat School, Ilwaco, Washington.

15. Unless otherwise noted, all quotes and material on Ryan are from Ryan, audiotaped interview with author, 29 January 2003, Station Cape Disappointment, Washington. Tape in author's files.

16. Other information on case comes from SAR folder, UCN 251, Station Cape Disappointment, Washington. Case folder obtained through a Freedom of Information Act request.
17. "Eric Forslund," *AFRAS Newsletter,* 3.
18. Ibid.
19. Anne Kifer, Secretary, AFRAS to author, e-mail, 14 December 2003.
20. All material on this case comes from SAR folder, UCN 236, Station Morro Bay, California. Case folder obtained through a Freedom of Information Act request. I wish to thank BMC Michael Saindon, officer in charge of Station Morro Bay, for his assistance in working with me on this case.
21. Hahn, "Coast Guard Rescues 4 Boaters."
22. Ibid.
23. Ibid.
24. Unless otherwise noted, all quoted material on Station Erie's rescue is found in SAR Incident Report Folder, UCN 059-03, located in the station's files. Folder was obtained through a Freedom of Information Act request. I am indebted to Chief Boatswain's Mate Jon Gagnon, officer in charge of Station Erie, for his help on this case.
25. Other U.S. Coast Guard personnel who played important roles in this case were, at Station Erie, Boatswain's Mate 2d Class Benjamin Heinze, the officer of the day, and communications watchstanders Boatswain's Mate 3d Class Jason Balmer, Boatswain's Mate 3d Class Melanie Schmidt, and Seaman John Bucaria. At Group Buffalo, Operations Specialist 1st Class Paul Angellilo and Group Communications Watchstander, Operations Specialist 3d Class Christopher Vilbrant. Information found in UCN 059-03.
26. Hahn, "Coast Guard Rescues 4 Boaters."

Chapter 14. Helicopters versus Gales

1. The *Gale Runner* case appeared in a different form in Noble, *Rescue of the Gale Runner.*
2. Quoted in Todd Lewan, "Into the Teeth of the Storm," *Reader's Digest,* June 1999, 103; "Incident Chronological Log," U.S. Coast Guard Air Station Sitka, Alaska. Obtained through the Freedom of Information Act (all material concerning this case from official U.S. Coast Guard records hereafter cited as La Conte case); "Northern Exposure," 38.

3. Quoted in Lewan, "Into the Teeth of the Storm," 101.

4. Ibid., 101–2.

5. "Northern Exposure," 38; Lewan, "Into the Teeth of the Storm," 103–4.

6. Walker, *Coming Back Alive,* 177–78. Walker's book is one of the most detailed books on a U.S. Coast Guard helicopter rescue and should be read by anyone interested in SAR.

7. Lewan, "Storm Gods and Heroes," pt. 2; *Seattle Post-Intelligencer,* December 29, 1998, p. B-1.

8. Quoted in Walker, *Coming Back Alive,* 178.

9. Ibid., 178–79.

10. Lewan, "Into the Teeth of the Storm," 104.

11. Quoted in Walker, *Coming Back Alive,* 180.

12. Quoted in Lewan, "Into the Teeth of the Storm," 104.

13. "Northern Exposure," 38.

14. Lewan, "Into the Teeth of the Storm," 104.

15. Walker, *Coming Back Alive,* 195.

16. Quoted in ibid., 192.

17. Walker, *Coming Back Alive,* 196.

18. La Conte case; "Northern Exposure," 39.

19. Quoted in "Northern Exposure," 39.

20. Walker, *Coming Back Alive,* 218.

21. Quoted in "Northern Exposure," 40.

22. Quoted in ibid., 41.

23. Ibid.

24. Walker, *Coming Back Alive,* 215–16.

25. "Northern Exposure," 41,

26. Quoted in Walker, *Coming Back Alive,* 225–26.

27. Quoted in ibid., 231.

28. Ibid., 227–30; Lewan, "Into the Teeth of the Storm," 105.

29. Quoted in "Northern Exposure," 42.

30. Walker, *Coming Back Alive,* 235.

31. Quoted in ibid.

32. "Northern Exposure," 42.

33. Quoted in ibid.

34. Ibid., 43.

35. The other crews and helicopters were as follows: Helicopter 6018—William Adickes, Daniel Molthen, Sean Witherspoon, and Richard Sansone; Helicopter 6029—David Durham, Russel Zullick, Chris Windnagle, and Arthur Thompson.

36. Quoted in "Northern Exposure," 43.

Epilogue

1. The percentage of people who serve at the stations is actually lower. The above numbers represent 416 people on active duty after 11 September 2001. Without the reservists, the number of actual active-duty people at the stations totaled 5,548. Numbers obtained from Lt. Bill Gibbons, Surfman Program Officer COMDT (G-OCS-1), U.S. Coast Guard Headquarters, Washington, D.C., to author, e-mail, 18 November 2003; Richard Schaefer, Office of Search and Rescue, U.S. Coast Guard Headquarters, Washington, D.C., to author, e-mail, 20 November 2003.

2. Of the 5,964 people serving at 188 small boat stations, 21 are officers, 33 are Chief Warrant Officers, and 5,908 are enlisted. These numbers include 416 reservists on active duty. Gibbons to author, 18 November 2003.

3. "Budget Statistics," www.uscgmil/hq/g-cp/comrel/factfile/index.htim.

4. As an example of lack of funding, on 23 March 2001, two U.S. Coast Guardsmen from Station Niagara, New York, drowned in the frigid waters of Lake Ontario. The investigation that followed found, among other items, that lack of funding failed to provide personal antiexposure equipment for each crew member. Investigation found that the crew had to share their equipment. The message outlining the final report of the investigation stated that the Office of Boat Forces in Headquarters would "advance funding efforts through the normal budget process to provide personal issue antiexposure suits and undergarments to each boat crew member at appropriate units." Furthermore, Capt. W. Russell Webster, U.S. Coast Guard (Ret.) stated in an e-mail that the "Niagara event caused G-O [Operations in Headquarters] to fast track the early acquisition of . . . [personal protection equipment] fleet wide by pumping additional monies into the system." While on active duty, Captain Webster was the president, Niagara MISHAP Analysis Board. Capt. W. Russell Webster to author, e-mail, 27 October 2003.

5. Personal observation and communication while in a 47-foot motor lifeboat in the Pacific Northwest. A former commanding officer of a station stated about crew communications aboard the 47-foot motor lifeboat: "Every mishap, every boat conference, every surfman conference, etc., the same request is made, the same determination of finding and fact is . . . we need crew comms [communications aboard the 47-footer]. G-OCS [Office of Boat Forces in Headquarters] has acknowledged and promised for 5 years now that they are developing a crew comm package. Guess what? I'm still waiting and there still is no package. . . . I asked G-OCS and they said they were getting closer. Bottom line is cost. A water hardened wireless system similar to what the SEALS have is approx[imately] $4K [thousand] a person." Source who does not wish to be identified to author, e-mail, 27 October 2003.

6. Goward, "Life-Saving Service," 52–56.

7. For a discussion of the disconnect, see Noble,"Unless There Was a Death," 64–69.

8. The two books on the modern stations are Noble, *Lifeboat Sailors* and Noble, *Rescue of the Gale Runner.* The autobiography is Webber, *Chatham.*

9. Paul J. Dupuis to author, e-mail, 21 April 2003.

10. CWO2 F. Scott Clendenin, interview with author, 18–19 March 1999, Station Yaquina Bay, Oregon.

11. BMCS Thomas Doucette, interview with author, 11–12 December 1996, Station Cape Disappointment, Washington.

12. Quoted in Noble, *Lifeboat Sailors,* 159.

13. Quoted in ibid., 209–10.

14. Quoted in Noble, *That Others Might Live,* vii.

Bibliography

Primary Sources

Columbia River Maritime Museum, Astoria, Oregon
  Coast Guard File
  Trinidad File

Evanston Historical Society, Evanston, Illinois
  Lawrence O. Lawson Files

Federal Records Center, Suitland, Maryland
  Station Log Books (Journals) for various stations and dates

Historian of the U.S. Coast Guard. U.S. Coast Guard Headquarters, Washington, D.C.

Disaster Files

  Marine Board of Investigation; Structural Failure of Tanker FORT MERCER off Cape Cod on 18 February 1952, with Loss of Life

  Marine Casualty Report OCEAN EXPRESS (Drilling Unit); Capsizing and Sinking in the Gulf of Mexico on 15 April 1976 with Loss of Life. Report No. USCG/61865. 1 June 1978.

  U.S. Coast Guard Board of Investigation, Serial A25/5097, 14 February 1961, Seattle, Washington. (*Mermaid* case.)

Subject Files

Records of the U.S. Coast Guard. RG 26. National Archives and Records
Administration, Washington, D.C.
"Miscellaneous, 1849–75," Box 1
Scrapbooks of the U.S. Life-Saving Service
Wreck Reports

U.S. Coast Guard SAR Incident Folders
Air Station Sitka, Alaska
Station Cape Disappointment, Washington
Station Erie, Pennsylvania
Station Morro Bay, California
Station Oregon Inlet, North Carolina

U.S. Coast Guard Station Scrapbooks
Station Humboldt Bay, California
Station Tillamook Bay, Oregon

Westport Maritime Museum, Westport, Washington
Some Coast Guard Rescues and Incidents from the Memoirs of
Hilman John Persson. C. 1977. Acc. 87-3-18/7.
Memoirs of Fridolph Persson. January 1977. Acc. 87-3-18/7.

Secondary Sources

AFRAS Newsletter. Arlington, Va.: Association for Rescue at Sea. Various
dates.

Baarslag, Karl. *Coast Guard to the Rescue.* New York: Farrar & Rinehart,
1936.

Barnett, J. Paul. "The Lifesaving Guns of David Lyle." *Wreck & Rescue:
The Journal of the U.S. Life-Saving Service Heritage Association* 5
(Summer 1997): 3–9.

Beard, Barrett Thomas. "Nineteen, Talk to Me!" U.S. Naval Institute
Proceedings 121 (August 1995): 66–71.

———. *Wonderful Flying Machine: A History of U.S. Coast Guard
Helicopters.* Annapolis: Naval Institute Press, 1996.

Bearss, Edwin C. "The 'Mirlo' Rescue." *North Carolina Historical
Review* 45 (October 1968): 384–98.

Bennett, Robert F. "The Lifesavers: 'For Those in Peril on the Sea.'" U.S.
Naval Institute *Proceedings* 102 (March 1976): 54–63.

———. *Surfboats, Rockets, and Carronades.* Washington, D.C.: GPO,
1976.

Dalton, J. W. *The Life Savers of Cape Cod.* Boston: Barta Press, 1902.

Davis, Rebecca Harding. "Life Saving Stations." *Lippincott's Magazine* 17 (March 1876): 301–10.

Earle, W. K. "A Saga of Ships, Men and the Sea: When Two Ships Foundered off Cape Cod, the Coast Guard Was Ready." *Coast Guard Magazine,* June 1952, 12–18.

Evans, Stephen H. *The United States Coast Guard, 1790–1915: With a Postscript: 1915–1949.* Annapolis: Naval Institute Press, 1949.

Flint, William. *Lightships of the United States Government: Reference Notes.* Washington, D.C.: Historian's Office, U.S. Coast Guard, 1989.

Frump, Robert. *Until the Sea Shall Free Them.* New York: Doubleday, 2002.

Galluzzo, John. "Big Shoes to Fill." *Wreck & Rescue: The Journal of the U.S. Life-Saving Service Heritage Association* 18 (Winter 2001): 4–8.

———. "Those Guys Got Plenty of Guts, Take It from Me: Hilman J. Persson and the Rescue of the Crew of the Trinidad." *Wreck & Rescue: The Journal of the U.S. Life-Saving Service Heritage Association* 17 (Fall 2001): 14–17.

Gibbs, Jim. *Pacific Graveyard.* Portland, Oreg.: Binfords & Mort, 1950.

———. *Shipwrecks of the Pacific Coast.* Portland, Oreg.: Binfords & Mort, 1957.

Goward, Dana A. "Life-Saving Service: Left in the Cold." U.S. Naval Institute *Proceedings* 125 (December 1999): 52–56.

Hahn, Tim. "Coast Guard Rescues 4 Boaters." *Erie (Pa.) Times-Review,* 9 July 2003.

Holland, Francis Ross, Jr. *America's Lighthouses: Their Illustrated History since 1716.* Brattleboro, Vt.: Stephen Green Press, 1972.

Howe, M. A. DeWolfe. *The Humane Society of the Commonwealth of Massachusetts: An Historical Overview.* Boston: Riverside Press, 1918.

Johnson, Robert Erwin. *Guardians of the Sea: History of the United States Coast Guard, 1915 to the Present.* Annapolis: Naval Institute Press, 1987.

Kaplan, H. R., and James F. Hunt. *This Is the Coast Guard.* Cambridge, Md.: Cornell Maritime Press, 1972.

Kimball, Sumner I. *Joshua James: Life-Saver.* Boston: American Unitarian Association, 1909.

————. *Organization and Methods of the United States Life-Saving Service . . . Read before the Committee on Life-Saving Systems and Devices, International Marine Conference, November 2, 1889.* Washington, D.C.: GPO, 1912.

Kroll, C. Douglas. *Commodore Ellsworth P. Bertholf: First Commandant of the U.S. Coast Guard.* Annapolis: Naval Institute Press, 2002.

Lester, Marianne. "When You're Raised Around the Water, You Don't See the Danger in It." *Navy Times* insert, *Times Magazine,* 17 May 1975, 6–7.

Lewan, Todd. "Into the Teeth of the Storm." *Reader's Digest,* June 1999, 98–107.

————. "Storm Gods and Heroes." *Seattle Post-Intelligencer,* 29–31 December 1998.

Means, Dennis R. "A Heavy Sea Running: The Formation of the U.S. Life-Saving Service, 1846–1878." *Prologue: Journal of the National Archives* 19, no. 4 (Winter 1987): 222–43.

Nalty, Bernard C., Dennis L. Noble, and Truman R. Strobridge, eds. *Wrecks, Rescues and Investigations: Selected Documents of the U.S. Coast Guard and Its Predecessors.* Wilmington, Del.: Scholarly Resources, 1978.

Noble, Dennis L. "End of an Era." *Wreck & Rescue: The Journal of the U.S. Life-Saving Service Heritage Association* 15 (Fall 2000): 15–18.

————. "Lawrence O. Lawson: An Extraordinary Keeper." *Wreck & Rescue: The Journal of the U.S. Life-Saving Service Heritage Association* 6, no. 1 (May 2003): 14–6.

————. *Lifeboat Sailors: Disasters, Rescues, and the Perilous Future of the Coast Guard's Small Boat Stations.* Washington, D.C.: Brassey's, 2000.

————. "Lifesaver," *Wreck & Rescue: The Journal of the U.S. Life-Saving Service Heritage Association* 5, no. 4 (February 2003): 8–11.

————. *The Rescue of the Gale Runner: Death, Heroism, and the U.S. Coast Guard.* Gainesville: University Press of Florida, 2002.

————. *That Others Might Live: The U.S. Life-Saving Service, 1878–1914.* Annapolis: Naval Institute Press, 1994.

———. "Unless There Was a Death," U.S. Naval Institute *Proceedings* 127 (December 2001): 64–69.

Noble, Dennis L., and T. Michael O'Brien. "Incident at Ashtabula." U.S. Naval Institute *Proceedings* 106 (October 1980): 128–29.

———. *A Legacy.* Washington, D.C.: U.S. Coast Guard, 1988.

———. *Southwest Pacific: A Brief History U.S Coast Guard Operations.* Washington, D.C.: U.S. Coast Guard, 1989.

———. "Soviets on a Shoestring," U.S. Naval Institute *Proceedings* 115 (October 1989): 140–141.

———. "That Others Might Live: The Saga of the U.S. Coast Guard." *American History Illustrated,* June 1977, 5–7, 37–43.

Noble, Dennis L., and Truman R. Strobridge. "You Have to Go Out." *Naval History* 3, no. 4 (Fall 1989): 12–20.

"Northern Exposure." *Rotor & Wing,* November 1999, 36–43.

O'Brien, T. Michael, and Dennis L. Noble, "Heroes on Ninety-three Cents a Day." *Inland Seas: Journal of the Great Lakes Historical Society* 33, no. 3 (Fall 1977): 192–205.

O'Connor, William D. *Heroes of the Storm.* Boston: Houghton, Mifflin, 1904.

Oleszewski, Wes. *Lighthouse Adventures: Heroes, Haunts and Havoc on the Great Lakes.* Gwinn, Mich.: Avery Color Studios, 1999.

Pearcy, Arthur. *U.S. Coast Guard Aircraft since 1916.* Annapolis: Naval Institute Press, 1991.

Scheina, Robert L. *A History of Coast Guard Aviation.* Washington, D.C.: Historian's Office, 1986.

———. *U.S. Coast Guard Cutters and Craft, 1946–1990.* Annapolis: Naval Institute Press, 1990.

———. *U.S. Coast Guard Cutters and Craft of World War II.* Annapolis: Naval Institute Press, 1982.

Schreiner, Samuel A. *Mayday! Mayday! The Most Exciting Missions of Rescue, Interdiction and Combat in the 200-year Annals of the U.S. Coast Guard.* New York: D. I. Fine, 1990.

Shanks, Ralph C., Jr., and Janetta Thompson Shanks. *Lighthouses and Lifeboats on the Redwood Coast.* San Anselmo, Calif.: Costano Books, 1978.

Shanks, Ralph C., Jr., Wick York, and Lisa Woo Shanks. *The U.S. Life-Saving Service: Heroes, Rescues and Architecture of the Early Coast Guard*. Petaluma, Calif.: Costano Books, 1996.

Stick, David. *Graveyard of the Atlantic: Shipwrecks of the North Carolina Coast*. Chapel Hill: University of North Carolina Press, 1952.

U.S. Coast Guard. *Deeds of Valor from the Annals of the U.S. Coast Guard*. Washington, D.C.: GPO, 1943.

——. *Register of the Commissioned and Warrant Officers and Cadets of the United States Coast Guard in the Order of Precedence*. Washington, D.C.: U.S. Coast Guard. Various years.

——. *The U.S. Coast Guard at War*. Vol. 14, *Assistance*. Washington, D.C.: Statistical Division and Historical Section, Public Information Division, U.S. Coast Guard, 1944–54.

U.S. Life-Saving Service. *Annual Report of the Operations of the United States Life-Saving Service for the Fiscal Year Ending June 30, 1876–1914*. Washington, D.C.: GPO, 1876–1914.

Van Dorn, William G. *Oceanography and Seamanship*. New York: Dodd, Mead, 1974.

Viola, Herman J., and Carolyn Margolis, eds. *Magnificent Voyagers: The U.S. Exploring Expedition, 1838–1848*. Washington, D.C.: Smithsonian Institution Press, 1985.

Walker, Spike. *Coming Back Alive*. New York: St. Martin's, 2001.

Waters, John M., Jr. "Finally the Twain Did Meet." Naval Aviation Museum *Foundation* 12 (Spring 1991): 92–99.

——. *Rescue at Sea*. New York: D. Van Nostrand, 1966.

Webber, Bernard C. *Chatham "The Lifeboatmen": A Narrative by a Seaman Recounting His Life in the Coast Guard at Chatham on the Southeast Corner of Cape Cod, Massachusetts*. Orleans, Mass.: Lower Cape Publishing, 1985.

Webster, W. Russell. "The *Pendelton* Rescue." U.S. Naval Institute *Proceedings* 127 (December 2001): 66–71.

Wilder, Kimberly. "I'm Gonna Die!" *Coast Guard*, July 2000, 19.

Wolff, Julius F., Jr. "One Hundred Years of Rescues: The Coast Guard on Lake Superior." *Inland Seas: The Quarterly Journal of the Great Lakes Historical Society* 31, no. 4 (Winter 1975): 265–75.

Index

ABOUT THE AUTHOR

Dennis L. Noble entered the U.S. Coast Guard in 1957 and retired in 1978 as a senior chief petty officer. He served at shore stations, including a lifeboat station, and in polar icebreakers, with six trips to the Arctic and two to the Antarctic. After retirement, he earned a Ph.D. in U.S. history from Purdue University. In 2003, Dr. Noble received the Columbia River Maritime Museum's Fellow of Maritime History, their highest honor for contributions to maritime history. He is one of only five people to receive this award from the museum. Noble is author of eleven previous books. He writes full time and lives in Sequim, Washington, with his wife, Loren, and a strange dog.